REAL LIFE ANTI-AGING HEALTH STRATEGIES

Lifestyle Habits to look your youngest,
achieve vitality, and sustain a sound mind

REAL LIFE ANTI-AGING HEALTH STRATEGIES

JACKLEINE SPRING

Published by Solid Ground House Publishing
Printed in the United States of America
Henderson, Nevada
SolidGroundHousePublishing.com

**SOLID
GROUND
HOUSE**
PUBLISHING
BOOKS THAT DIG DEEPER

Library of Congress Cataloging-in- Publication Data
Names: Spring, Jackleine
Title:REAL LIFE ANTI-AGING HEALTH STRATEGIES: Lifestyle Habits to look your youngest, achieve vitality, and sustain a sound mind / Jackleine Spring

Description: First Edition | Nevada: Solid Ground House Publishing

Identifiers: LCCN 9798999023209| ISBN (soft cover) 979-8-9990232-2-3 |
            ISBN (hard cover) 979-8-9990232-0-9 | ISBN (ebook) 979-8-9990232-1-6

Subject: Wellness strategies—Holistic. | Health.Classification

This book is dedicated to my best friend and husband–Mark

Who is always by my side ready and willing to try any of the health opportunities that come our way.

CONTENTS

PART 1
Fueling Youthfulness: Food Foundations

CHAPTER 1

Breakfast is the most important meal of the day

PART 2
Strategic Support: Supplements, Herbs & Detox

CHAPTER 5
Supplements

CHAPTER 6
The fast

PART 3
Movement & Daily Maintenance

CHAPTER 7
Motion

PART 4

PRELUDE

YOU DON'T HAVE TO LOOK OLDER
THAN YOU FEEL.

We were waiting for dinner one evening at a fine local eating house. The subtle echo of jazz fusion drifted through the air as I glanced around the room, casually people-watching. Clusters of individuals filled the tables around us, and a waiter passed by on his way to the next.

That's when I noticed her—a radiant woman with long dark hair ordering a drink. She looked effortlessly youthful, but there was wisdom in her eyes. The waiter asked to see her ID. I couldn't help but overhear. She was 55 years old. I was stunned. She looked decades younger. I wondered—did she feel as old as she looked? Or did she feel her age?

What was her secret? Was it what she ate? Something she used? What else could I be doing? I was already committed to being healthy, but I still felt the questions swirl. How old do we feel—and why?

That moment stuck with me. It was years ago, but I never forgot her. I was already deep into the health journey at the time, but that encounter gave me another layer to think about.

Now, many years later, I'm still aging—like we all are. But I truly believe: you feel as old as you look.

MY BACK STORY

HEALTH AS A WAY OF LIFE

Healthy is beautiful. But it's not something you just do—it's a way of life. I've spent years putting health strategies at the center of my choices, whether it's meal planning, troubleshooting an ailment, or refining the ingredients that go on and in my body. I always aim for the most natural, unprocessed path. Our world is full of contaminants and toxins that chip away at our energy, clarity, and youth. I've made it my mission to fight back—daily, intentionally, and naturally.

People often tell me, "You're so lucky you never get sick," or "You don't even seem to age." But luck isn't the reason. It takes conscious, consistent work to protect yourself from the overload we live in today. This book is a result of that work—a collection of practical tools, routines, and real strategies I've used to stay vibrant and clear-minded.

Like you, I've had to navigate conflicting advice. Books often made sense. But once I started reading magazines, the confusion began. One source praised soy. Another condemned it. For a while, the contradictions felt overwhelming. But I chose to use the chaos as motivation—to experiment, observe, and find out what actually worked for me.

This book isn't based on theory. It's built on real experiences—wins, flops, and the slow process of discovery. I've had to ask myself over and over: Is this a detox reaction or a negative one? Is this new supplement helping or hurting? Through trial, journaling, and curiosity, I started to assemble a health philosophy that works.

Let me give you a snapshot of how this all came to be.

A LOOK BACK

I was born in 1970 and raised in Michigan. In the '80s, we drank water right from the tap or garden hose—and didn't think twice. Back then, "health" didn't feel complicated. Now it seems like everyone's drinking out of plastic bottles and questioning every bite. Water is still my main drink today, and my husband and I quit alcohol completely in 2017. We live simply—black coffee in the morning, hot tea at night. Even when dining out, I ask for hot water with lemon or iced green tea. We don't overcomplicate it.

As a child, I had a healthy start. I remember my grandmother giving me chewable vitamin C during our visits to Detroit. She fasted at times too—even once doing a grape fast for a month. She made it to her 90s. I'm hopeful some of that longevity runs in the family.

In my teens, I got my first antibiotic for a sinus infection. Years later, everyone around me seemed to have chronic sinus issues. Five of us at work ended up getting sinus surgery. After rounds of antibiotics, my microbiome was wrecked. For my sinuses, I tried everything for relief—and finally found peroxide ear rinses to be incredibly effective. I used them daily for over a decade. Just be cautious—especially if there's a chance of a ruptured eardrum, as we learned the hard way with my husband!

NAVIGATING FOOD FADS

I've gone through the "healthy" trends—from soy meats and baked tofu to vegetarian weeks with limited protein. Looking back, I believe we did more harm than good with those choices. The labels were long, the ingredients were processed, and something just felt off. Then I met a woman at church who ate simple, classic meals—meatballs, spaghetti—not even organic. Yet she and her husband were healthy and slim. That encounter shifted my thinking. We started eating regular meals again—meats, sides, all home-cooked.

Then came Nourishing Traditions by Sally Fallon. That book changed everything. It opened the door to ancestral nutrition, fermented foods, and nutrient-dense recipes. I dove headfirst—fermenting carrots, ginger, beets, marmalade, and even lemonade. I made my own whey and used it in everything. But even good things can go too far. Eventually, I developed irritation. Our digestion got out of balance. Whoever heard of too much lactobacillus? We had to stop everything, reset our stomachs, and get back to simplicity. Apple cider vinegar came back in. The ferments went out. Balance was key.

HARD LESSONS, REAL WINS

In my late 40s and early 50s, I battled neuritis and cystitis. Doctors kept telling me I was "fine"—but I was in pain and desperate for answers. I kept trying new supplements. Some helped. Eventually, I found the ones that made a real difference.

Cholesterol became another chapter. I'd been craving butter for years, and I didn't hold back. That led me to explore the carnivore community—and discover how fats support hormones, sleep, and mental clarity. I now mix olive oil with butter. Sometimes I take a spoonful of fat before bed or if I wake in the night. It's calming and antimicrobial. We used to bake with coconut oil, but when our cholesterol hit 300, we eased off and saw it drop quickly. That showed me how powerful our food choices really are.

LIVING IT EVERY DAY

Now, past 50, I'm proud to say that my husband and I feel incredible. We're not slowing down. Our two dogs are sixteen and still run like pups.

We eat home-cooked meals, oven-baked chicken, burger, rice, vegetables, and simple sides. No fluff. No trends. Just real food and steady routines.

This book isn't about perfection. It's about finding what actually works—and sticking with it. You'll see that reflected in the strategies ahead. They're clean, realistic, and rooted in real life.

ONE LAST WORD BEFORE WE BEGIN

I'm not a doctor, and nothing in this book should be seen as medical advice. This is for informational and entertainment purposes only. What I share here is the result of my own research, trial and error, and commitment to living well.

These are the strategies that have worked for me and my family. And now, I'm passing them on to you.

INTRODUCTION

I've spent most of my life using health as a daily compass—constantly making decisions with one question in mind: Will this help me feel my best and stay strong as I age? That's always been the goal. Not to live forever—but to live well. To stay sharp, feel energized, and remain physically capable for as long as possible. Who doesn't want to be pain-free, mobile, and full of vitality—whether it's for work, recreation, or just getting through a full day with ease?

We all want to keep our spark. That glow. That energy that makes us feel alive and ready—not sidelined by exhaustion or stiffness. And I believe we can. That's what this book is about: preserving your youthfulness, not just in how you look, but in how you move, think, and show up for your life.

It doesn't matter where you live or what you do for a living—you can be that person who doesn't give up on health. Who keeps improving. Who stays in the game.

I'm committed to choosing the least toxic options available for anything life throws at me—from what I eat to what I put on my skin. That includes skincare, supplements, household products, and the food I serve to my husband and even our dogs. We eat from-scratch meals and read every label. If a product has more than one or two ingredients, we usually skip it. Clean eating has become our way of life. Simple. Intentional. And surprisingly powerful—even while living in the middle of city culture.

Of course, we're not perfect. We've had our share of health challenges and setbacks. But we push through them and learn from every experience. Many of the remedies we've tried have helped us stay strong, while others missed the mark. That's all part of the journey. And that's what I'm sharing here—a real, personal narrative about what's worked for us and what hasn't.

This book is built around strategies for clean food, active living, smart supplementation, detox, topical care, and mental clarity. Some things might surprise you. Others might be refreshingly simple. My hope is that these strategies help you build a lifestyle that makes you feel more alive, more youthful, and more grounded—no matter your age.

PART 1

FUELING YOUTHFULNESS: FOOD FOUNDATIONS

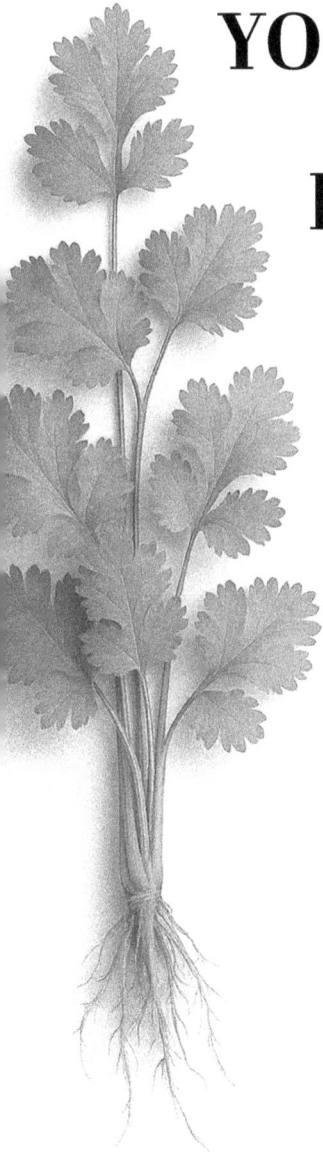

Chapter 1

BREAKFAST IS THE MOST IMPORTANT MEAL OF THE DAY

THIS IS WHERE YOUR ANTI-AGING ROUTINE TRULY BEGINS

Why how you start your morning
*shapes how young you **look and feel***

So many people just wake up and rush out the door—and I've never understood that. The morning hours are some of the most powerful in your day. This is when your body is most receptive to healing, energizing, and activating the systems that keep you youthful. Taking proper time in the morning isn't optional if your goal is long-term health, vitality, and a sound mind—it's foundational.

I view mornings as a time to intentionally activate the body: stimulate circulation, support digestive flow, and spark bile production to prep the system for nutrient absorption. Everything we do in the first few hours of the day influences how we feel for the next sixteen. That's why we cook from scratch, using whole, organic ingredients. There's a rhythm to it, and we've made it part of our lifestyle.

But health isn't just food—it's atmosphere, mindset, and connection. My husband and I start the day together, preparing breakfast and lunch not just for ourselves, but for our dogs too. It's a routine that's both grounding and uplifting. We create the environment we want to carry with us throughout the day. We play calming nature videos—birds, water, forest sounds—whatever feels right that morning. It sets the tone before the noise of the world creeps in.

These small habits aren't fluff. They are anti-aging strategies. They lower stress, regulate hormones, improve digestion, and protect your nervous system. Its physical and emotional alignment. It's movement and stillness. It's nourishment and intention.

Because the truth is, youthfulness doesn't begin with a product. It begins with a practice. And it starts right here—in your kitchen, your home, your morning.

COFFEE:
SIMPLE, STRONG, AND HEALTH-FOCUSED

One of the easiest, most powerful ways to start the morning right is with a cup of real black coffee. It's simple, it's classic, and when done right, it's a strategic tool for promoting energy, mental clarity, and cellular health.

Black coffee is naturally rich in antioxidants, compounds that protect the body against oxidative stress—the same stress that accelerates aging at the cellular level. It's been shown to support metabolism, brain function, and liver health—all critical systems for maintaining youthfulness and resilience.

We drink our coffee pure, without creams, sugars, or chemical-laden flavorings. Real coffee doesn't need dressing up. It's a natural stimulant that, in its raw form, energizes without the crash that comes from sugar-spiked beverages.

Unfortunately, today's coffee culture has drifted far from that simplicity. Many coffee shops have turned a natural drink into a processed dessert—filled with syrups, flavor shots, seed oils, artificial creamers, and enough sugar to sabotage the body's balance before the day even begins.

We once visited a popular coffee chain using a gift card and couldn't even find freshly brewed black coffee on the menu. It was a reminder that what's marketed as "coffee" today often has little to do with the real thing.

This is why we stick to what's real.

Simple black coffee.
Organic when possible.
Brewed fresh at home.

It's part of our anti-aging strategy: staying close to the earth, trusting what's pure, and choosing foods and habits that support sharpness, vibrancy, and strength—not just for today, but for years to come. Coffee, when respected in its natural form, becomes more than a beverage—it becomes a tool for sustaining youthfulness, energy, and a sound mind.

APPLE CIDER VINEGAR:
A DAILY CATALYST FOR VITALITY

Some strategies stand the test of time—and apple cider vinegar is one of them. This simple, powerful beverage has been a cornerstone of our morning routine for over twenty-five years, and it remains one of the most effective ways to activate digestion, support alkalinity, and prime the body for energy and youthfulness.

We start each day with a tablespoon of apple cider vinegar mixed into about six ounces of water. For years, we added a teaspoon of raw honey. Later we switched to real maple syrup for better mixing. Today, we prefer Manuka honey for its richer flavor and superior health benefits. (And yes—stirring with a wooden spoon, not metal, makes a difference!)

Apple cider vinegar works by stimulating natural acidity, encouraging bile production, and waking up the digestive system. It sets the stage for regularity, nutrient absorption, and balanced gut health—key foundations for looking and feeling youthful.

We never travel without it. Whenever we're exposed to unfamiliar foods or disrupted routines, apple cider vinegar is what keeps our digestion strong, our energy steady, and that bloated, sluggish feeling at bay. Once you experience the difference, you won't want to start a day—or a trip—without it.

The real power of apple cider vinegar isn't just in what it does—it's in doing it consistently. That's where lasting health, soundness of mind, and youthful vitality are built. "Once in a while" doesn't create real transformation. Daily action does. Consistency turns good ideas into results you can feel and see.

> ### APPLE CIDER VINEGAR
>
> • 1 six ounce cup water
> • 1 tablespoon apple cider vinegar
> • 1 teaspoon honey or maple syrup

This simple morning ritual is a direct investment in your digestion, your resilience, and your anti-aging strategy. It's not just about what you drink—it's about how you begin the day, every day.

Because a vibrant life isn't created by force—it's created by daily habits born out of real desire for health, strength, and clarity.

WHY APPLE CIDER VINEGAR SUPPORTS ANTI-AGING

▸ *Boosts digestion*
Stimulates natural stomach acidity and bile production for better nutrient absorption.

▸ *Supports gut health*
Creates a favorable environment for healthy bacteria, improving immunity and mental clarity.

▸ *Balances blood sugar*
Helps regulate insulin response, reducing spikes and crashes that accelerate aging.

▸ *Enhances detoxification*
Encourages liver and lymphatic system support, helping the body eliminate waste more efficiently.

▸ *Reduces bloating and inflammation*
Keeps digestion smooth and reduces the chronic inflammation that leads to premature aging.
▸ *Strengthens metabolic function*
Prepares the body for better energy utilization throughout the day.

Tip: Choose raw, unfiltered apple cider vinegar with the "mother" intact for the most potent health benefits.

CRANBERRY JUICE:
A DAILY DOSE OF CELLULAR POWER

For over twenty-five years, starting the day with our cranberry shooter has been one of our most reliable habits for protecting health, enhancing energy, and promoting youthful function from the inside out.

Unsweetened cranberry juice is a powerhouse. It's loaded with anti-oxidants, vitamins, minerals, and phytonutrients that support liver health, urinary tract balance, and powerful cellular defense against oxidative stress—the very stress that accelerates aging.

Our morning formula is simple but highly strategic:
▸ About 4 ounces of unsweetened cranberry juice
▸ 1–2 tablespoons of lemon juice
▸ 1 tablespoon of high-quality olive oil (we prefer California Olive Ranch 100% California)
▸ 4000 mg of MSM (a sulfur compound vital for every cell in the body)

Sometimes we add sea kelp for natural iodine. Over the years, we've tweaked the mix slightly, but the cranberry base has stayed constant—and the results speak for themselves.

We originally adapted this habit from the book The Fat Flush Plan, where the author recommended sipping a diluted cranberry mixture throughout the day. We customized it into a morning powerhouse shot for a faster, cleaner boost—and it's been a staple ever since.

WHY THIS MORNING RITUAL MATTERS

This cranberry shot isn't just a drink—it's a targeted tool for:

> ### CRANBERRY JUICE SHOOTER
>
> - Four ounces unsweetened cranberry juice
> - 1-2 tablespoons fresh lemon juice
> - I scoop or 4000 mg MSM
> - 1 tablespoon organic extra virgin olive oil

- ▸ Supporting liver detoxification (your key organ for longevity)
- ▸ Improving digestive strength (critical for nutrient absorption and regularity)
- ▸ Flooding the body with antioxidants (which combat skin aging and internal stress)
- ▸ Alkalizing the system (helping balance inflammatory patterns)

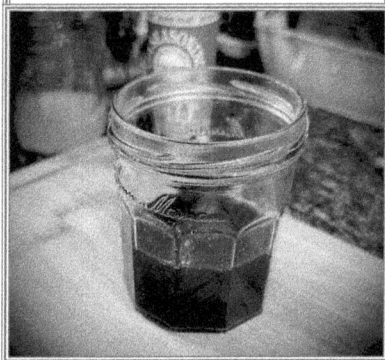

Over time, this ritual promotes stronger digestion, better cellular hydration, more efficient detox, and a lighter, more vibrant feeling throughout the body.

Whether you start this habit to restore health or to maintain it long-term, it's one of the most efficient ways to keep your internal systems young, clear, and high-functioning.

CONSISTENCY IS THE SECRET.

The best strategies for anti-aging are the simple ones you do every day without fail—where nourishment becomes a rhythm, not a reaction.

BUILDING THE FOUNDATION: MINERALS AND MORNING HEALTH ESSENTIALS

Strengthening the body's core systems to sustain youthfulness and vitality

UNREFINED SEA SALT: THE MINERAL-RICH ESSENTIAL YOU CAN'T AFFORD TO MISS

When it comes to foundational health strategies, minerals are non-negotiable—and salt is one of the easiest, most powerful ways to supply your body with what it needs to thrive.

But not just any salt.
Not bleached, processed, chemical-laden table salt.
Real salt. Natural salt. Mineral salt.

We've used Celtic sea salt exclusively for over twenty-five years. It's distinctly different from commercial salts, starting with its natural light gray color—a visible sign of its rich trace mineral content. Unlike refined table salts, which are stripped of nutrients and often laced with additives like anti-caking agents, Celtic sea salt delivers a broad spectrum of minerals in their natural, bioavailable form.

WHY MINERAL-RICH SALT SUPPORTS ANTI-AGING AND VITALITY

- Balances electrolytes naturally, keeping hydration and nerve function optimized
- Supplies critical trace minerals that support thyroid health, metabolism, and immune resilience
- Enhances digestion by stimulating natural enzyme production

- Promotes healthy blood pressure regulation when used properly with a clean diet

We cook all of our meals with Celtic sea salt, and we never hesitate to add a little more to taste. Unlike synthetic salts, real sea salt enhances the quality of food while supporting the body's natural mineral stores—key for maintaining vibrant energy and clear thinking as you age.

Some recommend drinking salt water first thing in the morning to boost mineral absorption. I've tried small amounts—about half a teaspoon diluted in water—but we get enough from the generous seasoning of our home-cooked meals, making it unnecessary for us right now.

A REAL-LIFE TESTIMONY: SALT AND RECOVERY

Several years ago, during a particularly rough bout of illness, I watched firsthand how Celtic sea salt made a rapid difference. After struggling with hydration and seeing oxygen levels dip unusually low, a simple teaspoon of Celtic sea salt in warm water brought immediate recovery. My oxygen numbers bounced back almost instantly.

Coincidence? Maybe.

But in our house, we believe the body recognizes what's real—and real minerals make a real difference.

Even our dogs benefit from Celtic sea salt in their meals. They love it, and I love knowing they're getting pure minerals to support their health naturally.

When it comes to maintaining strength, cellular function, and energy with age, Celtic sea salt isn't optional—it's essential.

HOW UNREFINED SEA SALT SUPPORTS ANTI-AGING

Mineral power for youthfulness, energy, and resilience

Core Benefits:
- Boosts hydration naturally by balancing electrolytes
- Strengthens the thyroid with trace minerals like iodine and selenium

- Promotes efficient digestion by stimulating enzyme production
- Enhances adrenal health and supports stress resilience
- Protects nerve function and cognitive clarity through mineral balance
- Supports healthy blood pressure when paired with a clean, unprocessed diet

Tip for Best Results: Choose unrefined, sun-dried sea salt that still retains its natural moisture and trace mineral richness.

Avoid overly processed "sea salts" that have been bleached or chemically altered.

IODINE:
THE TRACE MINERAL
THAT PROTECTS YOUTHFULNESS

When it comes to long-term vitality, few nutrients are as overlooked—and as critical—as iodine. This trace mineral is essential for thyroid health, hormone regulation, cellular energy, and mental sharpness. Without adequate iodine, the body's internal engine slows down, setting the stage for fatigue, weight gain, brain fog, hair thinning, and accelerated aging.

For years, we tried to meet our iodine needs naturally by adding sea kelp to our cranberry shooter. While sea kelp is a valuable food source, it simply couldn't supply the amount of iodine we needed to support full thyroid function. To get the ideal daily dose, you would need to consume large amounts of seaweed consistently—a challenge for most people.

That's when we transitioned to Lugol's iodine, a concentrated form of iodine that's been trusted for over a century.

We started looking into iodine for a couple of reasons. We were really into cabbage for years. We chopped it up and stir fried it on the stove with some olive oil and apple cider vinegar. Then we started making coleslaw homemade. It was pretty much prepared the same way. We ate it about four times a week. What could be wrong with cabbage? It's so good for you. Right? Well I guess cabbage and cruciferous vegetables have goitrogens. They affect your thyroid. My dogs love cabbage. They were getting it every day in their dinners. My dog and I ended up with some thyroid symptoms. My dog had a huge growth on her back. I had neck symptoms and my hair was so thin. We started taking some iodine.

HOW WE SUPPLEMENT WITH IODINE
We started slowly, adding just one or two drops to a small splash of coffee in a pottery shot glass each morning. Over time, we gradually increased to a comfortable dose based on how we felt and how our bodies responded.

(Everyone's needs are different—always research and adjust carefully. I highly recommend Dr. David Brownstein's work on iodine for an excellent foundation. Besides his YouTube channel having a plethora of information, I read his book on iodine. The title is 'Iodine: Why you need it, why you can't live without it').

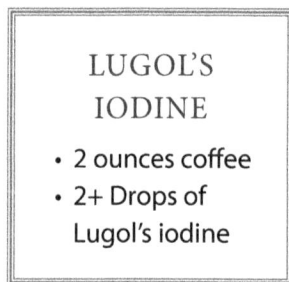

> ### LUGOL'S IODINE
> - 2 ounces coffee
> - 2+ Drops of Lugol's iodine

The results were undeniable:
- My energy levels lifted almost immediately.
- Chronic neck tightness and thyroid sensitivity disappeared.
- Hair began to regain its fullness and strength.
- Even our dog, who had developed thyroid-related tumors, showed visible improvement after being supplemented with a few drops daily—her tumors shrank significantly over a few months.

Iodine wasn't just a "supplement"—it became a cornerstone of protecting our vitality, clarity, and resilience as we age.

- Protects thyroid function, keeping metabolism strong and steady
- Promotes hormone balance, supporting smoother energy and mood regulation
- Enhances cognitive clarity, preventing mental fatigue and fog
- Strengthens immune resilience through cellular repair and detox pathways
- Supports healthy hair, nails, and skin—key visible markers of youth

We live in a time where iodine deficiency is widespread, thanks to depleted soils, processed foods, and chemical exposures.

If you're serious about longevity, energy, and maintaining a youthful, sound mind, iodine supplementation can be a powerful part of your anti-aging strategy. Natural, simple, and life-changing—that's the power of getting back to the essentials your body truly needs.

Tip for Best Results: Use a trusted iodine source like Lugol's solution. Start with small doses and increase slowly based on your body's feedback.

BACK TO THE BREAKFAST TABLE

Why we chose eggs, apples, and real food over processed trends

When it comes to preserving youthfulness and building lasting vitality, the first meal of the day matters more than most people realize. It's not just about eating—it's about fueling your body at the cellular level, setting up your hormones, metabolism, and digestion to work with you, not against you, for the rest of the day.

One of the biggest shifts we made early on was ditching processed cereals and commercial breads in favor of real, whole foods—starting with pasture-raised eggs and organic apples.

Letting Go of Cereal:
THE MORNING SHIFT THAT CHANGED EVERYTHING

Not long after we got married, I came across a bold recommendation in The Fat Flush Plan: eat eggs every day for breakfast.

It sounded simple, but for us it meant a real lifestyle shift. My husband had been a lifelong cereal eater. For years, like many Americans, he had answered the siren call of the cereal aisle—lured by decades of marketing that sold processed grains as "the healthy breakfast." And old habits die hard. At first, he'd eat his eggs with a side of cereal—trying to do both. I get it. That's what conditioning looks like.

But here's the truth: cereal is just processed filler—stripped of nutrients, pumped with sugar, fortified with synthetic vitamins, and often preserved with questionable additives like BHT. We've been fed the illusion that it's convenient, balanced, and even necessary. But it's not. It's a cleverly packaged product masquerading as health food.

And then there's the milk. First we gave up real food, and now we're giving up real milk, too? These milk impostors—soy, almond, oat—are just ultra-processed residue dressed up as wellness. They're not nourishing. They're not whole. Most are packed with gums, fillers, and inflammatory oils. I say drink real milk—from real cows—and make it whole milk while you're at it.

If I'm going to have something sweet in the morning, I'd rather make it myself: something warm, simple, and digestible—like a homemade muffin with clean ingredients I can pronounce. Real food. Not boxed.

Eventually, we gave up cereal completely—and we've never looked back. Breakfast is now a grounding meal: eggs, cheese, and fruit. A homemade pastry. It fuels us. It lasts.

Processed foods age you. Real foods build you.

Let go of the cereal—and watch what shifts.

EGGS:
A NUTRIENT-DENSE POWERHOUSE

Eggs are one of nature's most perfect foods. They deliver highly bioavailable protein, essential fatty acids, B vitamins, choline for brain health, and important fat-soluble nutrients—all of which are critical for maintaining youthful skin, strong metabolism, hormone balance, and cognitive sharpness.

Real food gives you real building blocks for health. Processed foods give you false fullness and hidden depletion.

APPLES:
FIBER, ACIDITY, AND NATURAL ENERGY

To balance the richness of the eggs, we added organic apples to our morning plate.

We slice one apple and share it. A few bites is enough to offer:

- ‣ Natural fruit sugars for quick, clean energy
- ‣ Fiber to promote healthy digestion and regularity
- ‣ Acidity that supports gut health and metabolic function

We stick to organic apples because non-organic varieties tend to be mealy, lacking flavor and acidity—and laden with pesticide residues. Our favorites are Honeycrisp, Cosmic Crisp, SugarBee, and green varieties—but any fresh, organic apple carries that same refreshing vitality.

Along with eating the apple, I usually add some bananas to our morning fruit plate. Can't go wrong with a banana straight out of the peel God put it in. Delish. And of course, our dogs get a few apple slices too—keeping the morning routine complete for the whole household.

BUILDING A BREAKFAST THAT FUELS YOUTH

As we moved away from cereal culture and into a more nourishing rhythm, our breakfast evolved into something truly rejuvenating. Eggs were the foundation—but what we built on top made all the difference.

I started experimenting with fresh herbs like parsley and cilantro—and now they're a daily staple. Just a couple sprigs, finely chopped and sprinkled over warm eggs, and the whole dish transforms. Not only do they taste incredibly fresh, but they also support detox, aid digestion, fight inflammation, and even freshen breath. These green herbs aren't just garnish—they're daily medicine.

I actually find that breakfast is the easiest time to incorporate herbs like this. By evening, routines can get busy and palates shift. But first thing in the morning? The herbs are energizing and bright. They pair beautifully with eggs and set a clean tone for the day.

> ## TWO FRIED EGGS
> - 1 tbsp organic butter
> - 1 tablespoon olive oil (to fry eggs)
> - 1-2 pasture raised eggs (per person)
> - 1 teaspoon organic chopped parsley
> - 1 teaspoon chopped organic cilantro
> - 1/2 1 slice provolone cheese
> - ground Cayenne pepper

We also add a dash of cayenne or other hot spices to kickstart circulation and support digestion. Our spice shelf has become a mini apothecary: ground Cayenne, Habanero, smoked Serrano, Thai chili powder. Just a pinch wakes up the metabolism and gets the blood flowing.

And let's not forget a drizzle of high-quality fat—like grass-fed butter, a little cold-pressed olive oil, or some coconut oil. These fats not only help absorb fat-soluble vitamins but also keep the meal satiating and skin-friendly. Healthy fats are your anti-aging allies.

Sometimes we'll even melt a little provolone cheese over the eggs for richness and comfort. It's clean, satisfying, and deeply nourishing.

Honestly, I'm surprised more restaurants don't offer herbs as a standard egg topping. If I ever opened a café, fresh herbs would be a given.

This is breakfast that works with your body, not against it. Youthful energy starts in the morning—with real food, real fat, and a little heat.

WHY REAL BREAKFAST FOODS PRESERVE YOUTHFULNESS

The nutrients your body needs to stay energized, resilient, and sharp.

CORE BENEFITS
- Eggs:
  Complete protein, choline for brain health, fat-soluble vitamins for skin, hormones, and metabolism
- Organic Apples:
  Natural sugars for clean energy, fiber for digestive health, and antioxidants to support cellular repair
- Fresh Herbs (Parsley & Cilantro):
  Detoxifiers that aid liver function, boost digestion, and freshen breath naturally
- Real Fats (Butter, Olive Oil, Coconut oil):
  Stabilize hormones, fuel brain cells, and support healthy skin and joint flexibility
- Hot Spices (Cayenne, Ghost Pepper, Thai Chili):
  Stimulate circulation, enhance digestion, and naturally elevate metabolic rate.

WHY THIS BREAKFAST STRATEGY MATTERS

This isn't about feeling stuffed. It's about feeling satisfied, energized, and mentally sharp without the crash or inflammation that comes from processed foods.

Fullness slows you down.
Satisfaction fuels you forward.

Breakfast becomes more than a meal—it becomes part of your anti-aging strategy, strengthening the very systems that keep you looking and feeling your best: digestion, metabolism, hormonal balance, and cognitive vitality.
We're not just feeding ourselves for today.
We're building our future health, one real meal at a time.

THE FATS THAT FEED YOU

Why real fats are essential for youthful energy, sharp thinking, and long-term vitality

For years, mainstream health advice demonized fat. But real science—and real life—prove otherwise: Healthy fats are not only essential—they are foundational if you want to look younger, feel stronger, and maintain mental clarity as you age.
Over the years, we've explored a wide range of natural fats, all rooted in one principle:
Stick to what's real. Stick to what your body was designed to recognize.
In our kitchen, we use:
- Pasture-raised butter
- Olive oil (preferably single-origin and cold-pressed)
- Organic coconut oil

- Beef tallow, lamb tallow
- Duck fat
- Pork lard, leaf lard

Most of our tallows and specialty fats come from trusted sources where the focus is purity, not processing.

WHY REAL FATS ARE ANTI-AGING ALLIES
- Support hormone production (critical for metabolism, skin health, and emotional resilience)
- Strengthen brain cell membranes, boosting cognitive function and mental sharpness
- Protect the skin from within, preserving elasticity and hydration
- Lower systemic inflammation, a root driver of aging and chronic disease
- Stabilize blood sugar, preventing insulin spikes and crashes that accelerate aging.

OLIVE OIL THAT WORKS

People often say not to fry with olive oil—but we've always used it for eggs without issue. The real secret? Quality. Most store-bought "olive oils" are diluted with cheap seed oils—even when the label doesn't admit it. That's why I stick with California Olive Ranch.

Their Global Blend is affordable and great for cooking, while their 100% California version is next-level: clean, light, and perfect for raw uses like coleslaw, dressings, and sauces. It's more delicate, so we save it for when flavor and freshness matter most.

When it's the real deal, olive oil becomes a powerful anti-aging ally. Cold-pressed, high-quality olive oil supports:
- Heart health and cholesterol balance
- Blood sugar regulation and healthy weight management

- Reduced inflammation linked to arthritis and chronic illness
- Improved digestion and nutrient absorption
- Cellular protection and long-term resilience through antioxidants

But here's what matters most: it's real food—not a synthetic oil made in a lab.

That's why we stay away from hydrogenated oils, margarine, seed oils, and anything industrial. These fake fats may look innocent, but they quietly disrupt hormones, strain the liver, and accelerate aging on a cellular level.

Even with real ingredients, quality varies by brand. That's why sourcing matters. I trust that every fat we use in our kitchen—from tallow to olive oil—is doing something good for our health, not sabotaging it.

A wise doctor once said:

"Fat-soluble nutrients are found in fat."

If you avoid real fats, you miss the natural delivery system for some of the most powerful anti-aging compounds your body needs to thrive.

Elizabeth Bright, and her book Good Fat is Good for Women: Menopause is one I highly recommend—it's informative and eye-opening.

The idea that fat is bad for us has been one of the biggest nutritional deceptions of our time. The truth is, real fats—like butter, cream, coconut oil, tallow, lard, and olive oil—are foods our bodies were designed to recognize. They're made by nature, not by a factory. There's no need for margarine or hydrogenated oils trying to impersonate them.

I was starting to believe the tides were finally turning. But then I had a conversation with a younger colleague who proudly told me he uses margarine because he thinks it's the healthier choice. It was a reminder: the seed oil narrative is still alive and well.

Artificial oils are everywhere. They fill the majority of packaged foods people consume daily. Even if people have heard they're harmful, many keep eating them—for the sake of convenience or because they've just gotten used to it.

Choosing real fats isn't just a preference.
It's a health strategy—one that will show up in your energy, your skin, your mental sharpness, and your resilience for years to come.

"Fat-soluble nutrients are found in fat."
Choosing real fats isn't a preference—
it's a health strategy.

WHY HEALTHY FATS ARE ANTI-AGING POWERHOUSES

Fuel your body, sharpen your mind, and protect your youth

CORE BENEFITS
- Support hormone production
  Vital for metabolism, energy, and mood regulation
- Streghten cognitive function
  Nourish brain cells and improve mental clarity
- Enhance skin vitality
  Preserve moisture, elasticity, and a youthful glow
- Reduce inflammation
  Calm the chronic inflammation that accelerates aging
- Stabilize blood sugar
  Prevent insulin spikes that damage tissues and speed aging
- Boost nutrient absorption
  Help absorb fat-soluble vitamins A, D, E, and K for total body health

REAL PASTRIES, REAL INGREDIENTS

How homemade simplicity supports youthfulness, digestion, and lasting vitality

Eating for vitality doesn't mean giving up the foods you love. It means redefining them—stripping away processed shortcuts and bringing back real ingredients your body recognizes, digests, and uses to maintain energy, mental clarity, and youthful resilience. Pastries are no exception.

In our home, they're not store-bought sugar bombs or processed flour concoctions. They're homemade treats, made from scratch, with simple, pure ingredients—foods that fuel rather than fog the body.

Most store-bought versions are packed with preservatives, seed oils, and synthetic additives. But when you make your own using real butter, organic flour, and pasture-raised eggs, they become a source of both joy and nourishment—something your body actually wants.

HOW OUR BREAKFAST PASTRIES CAME TO LIFE
A homemade tradition with anti-aging intention

Even back in high school, I had a soft spot for toast and berry preserves. There was something comforting about the ritual—the warmth, the fruit, the slight sweetness. But once I began to really understand how commercial breads and refined ingredients disrupt digestion, spike insulin, and lead to sluggish mornings, I made a change.

I gave up store-bought bread—and even homemade yeast breads—for good. No matter how "clean" I made it, bread left me feeling heavy and bloated. That full, stuffed feeling isn't nourishment—it's overload.

But I wasn't about to give up the joy of a little morning sweet. So I created something new.

That's how our real-food breakfast pastries were born: homemade, intentionally crafted, and deeply satisfying without the crash.

Here's how we make them:

- Organic, unbleached flour
- Pasture-raised butter and eggs
- Natural, unprocessed sweeteners like organic cane sugar or a touch of maple syrup
- No mixes, no additives, no seed oils

We batch-bake our pastries and freeze them. Each morning, we warm one gently on the stove—a little finishing touch after a protein-rich breakfast. It's the perfect companion to black coffee and doesn't weigh us down or undo the work of our clean start.

This isn't about denial—it's about real indulgence made with real ingredients. It's about knowing what's in your food and how it makes you feel—today, and in the long run.

Anti-aging isn't about restriction. It's about intentional nourishment. And yes, you can have your pastry and glow, too.

WHAT'S ON OUR PASTRY MENU?
- Chocolate-drizzled macadamia nut scones
- Molasses scones
- Simple butter biscuits
- Shortbread topped with real fruit preserves
- Blueberry streusel cake
- Homemade pancakes (from scratch, no prefab mixes)

Less Is More:
LEARNING TO BE SATISFIED

Just because the ingredients are real doesn't mean we eat endlessly. We split pastries. A couple bites is all we need. Fullness isn't the goal—satisfaction is. Feeling satisfied means you're nourished and energized, not bogged down or bloated. Too often, people confuse being full with being fueled. We've been asked,

"How do you get full from that?"—but we're not trying to get full. We're trying to feel good.

There's a huge difference between being satisfied and being stuffed. Fullness drags you down—mentally and physically. Satisfaction lifts you up, fuels energy, sharpens focus, and preserves your lightness throughout the day.

HOMEMADE MEANS HEALTHIER, LIGHTER, SMARTER

Because we control every ingredient, our pastries feel light, digest cleanly, and don't leave us bogged down.

We use simple substitutions that support digestion.

I make homemade buttermilk by mixing 1 tablespoon of apple cider vinegar into milk before adding it to the batter.

We tried alternative flours like buckwheat and spelt, but even those

> ### HOMEMADE BUTTERMILK
> • 1 tablespoon apple cider vinegar
> • 1/2 to 1 cup whole milk
> Let sit minimum 5-10 minutes to thicken.
> Use immediately

"healthier" versions caused weight gain over time. Once we stopped making those breads, the weight came right off. That's why we stick to the basics—flour, butter, milk, eggs—and keep our portions small and satisfying

WHY HOMEMADE PASTRIES MATTER FOR ANTI-AGING
- Support digestion with real foods the body can easily process
- Avoid chemical additives and preservatives that age cells and burden detox pathways
- Prevent blood sugar spikes and crashes that damage collagen, insulin sensitivity, and brain function
- Cultivate daily joy without sacrificing metabolic stability or mental sharpness

This isn't about deprivation.

It's about choosing foods that work for you, not against you.

It's about savoring real flavors, honoring your digestion, and staying aligned with the rhythms that build youthfulness, vibrancy, and long-term strength.

Homemade matters. Real food matters.
How you feel afterward matters.

FROM-SCRATCH SIMPLICITY

Where breakfast sets the tone for your whole day

This is how I start my day: with intention, real food, and ingredients that make me feel alive.

We might shop at the grocery store, but we treat it like farm-to-table living. We stick to the perimeter—where the food is fresh, whole, and recognizable. That means produce, quality eggs, dairy, and meats. We avoid the aisles full of artificial creations: no GMOs, no synthetic meats, no "meat glue," and no chemically engineered stand-ins pretending to be food.

We keep our meals centered on foods that are as close to their original form as possible—foods your body actually recognizes, digests, and uses. When you eat this way consistently, something shifts. Your palate resets. Processed foods lose their pull, and you start to crave what's clean. You feel the clarity. You want more of that energy, that lightness, that glow.

Our mornings are simple but satisfying. We build a nourishing breakfast—high-quality protein, natural fats, and a little sweet touch. It's not overdone, but it's beautiful. Thoughtfully portioned, deeply enjoyable, and supportive of our health goals.

We prepare it together. While we're making breakfast, we're also assembling lunches—so there's always a few moving parts. Everyone helps. It becomes a rhythm.

And we're not the only ones at the table.

Just as we finish our morning meal, it's time for the dogs to eat too. They've been patiently waiting—and their breakfast is just as intentional.

WHOLE HEALTH INCLUDES THE WHOLE FAMILY: DOGS INCLUDED

Fresh, real foods to nourish vitality—for us and our dogs

In our home, health isn't just a human pursuit—it's a family lifestyle. And that includes our dogs.

Their morning routine mirrors ours: built on real food, clean ingredients, and thoughtful care. We believe that just like us, dogs thrive on foods that are close to nature—foods their bodies understand and actually benefit from. That's how we start their day: intentionally, simply, and with love.

MORNING SNACKS: FRESH, CRUNCHY, AND SIMPLE

Every morning begins with a hand-fed treat—usually sugar snap peas or snow peas. These are small, crisp, and satisfying. They're:
- Rich in fiber
- Full of gentle, plant-based vitamins and minerals
- Easy on digestion and easy to portion

This ritual might seem small, but it creates connection. It sets the tone for a calm, fulfilled morning—for both them and us. It's a shared rhythm of wellness.

THE HEART OF THEIR BREAKFAST

For over sixteen years, our dogs have started their mornings with a fried egg—lightly cooked, and topped with the same fresh herbs we use ourselves: parsley and cilantro.

These herbs are more than garnish. They:
▸ Naturally freshen breath
▸ Support digestion
▸ Provide gentle detox
▸ Offer antimicrobial and antiviral benefits
▸ Help prevent nutrient-seeking behaviors like grass eating

MORNING NOURISHMENT FOR THE DOGS

Hand-Fed Start (They love this part)
• 4 sugar snap peas

• 3 small cubes of cooked chicken

Their Real Food Bowl
• 1 egg per dog
• Fresh parsley and cilantro
• Celtic sea salt (never table salt)
• Any daily supplements
  (e.g. MSM, hawthorn berry, burdock root powder)
• A pinch of sea kelp for thyroid and trace minerals

• A few apple slices to finish

Our dogs wait patiently as the eggs are prepared, their instincts tuned in to what real food smells like. This isn't kibble—it's nourishment their bodies recognize.

GENTLE SUPPLEMENTATION: TINY TOOLS, BIG BENEFITS

We keep their supplementation simple and natural, using the tiniest measuring tool—a "drop" spoon—to ensure precision without overload. Their core supports include:

- Burdock root, hawthorn berry, parsley, and cilantro (for gentle detox and cardiovascular support)
- MSM and diatomaceous earth (for joints, skin, and gut health)
- Iodine and sea kelp (for thyroid and trace mineral balance)
- Nutritional yeast and Celtic sea salt (for B vitamins and electrolytes)

We sprinkle powders over pre-cooked chicken or occasionally tuck tablets inside a small piece of real cheddar. It's easy, positive, and part of the routine.

APPLES, PANCAKES, AND HOMEMADE JOY

Just like us, our dogs enjoy a little morning sweetness. A few fresh apple slices with our breakfast? They get some, too.

And for their breakfast treat, we share homemade mini pancakes, cut into tiny one-inch bites. No artificial treats, no mass-produced snacks. Just real, clean food from our kitchen to their bowl.

Kibble is available in small bowls, but it's rarely touched. Over 90% of their diet comes from fresh food—the kind that builds strong bodies, soft coats, calm digestion, and lifelong resilience.

REAL FOOD BUILDS REAL VITALITY

Our dogs' health reflects the same truth we live by:

The closer you stay to nature, the stronger your body will be.

Eggs, herbs, peas, apples—these aren't just ingredients. They're part of a life rhythm that honors vitality, connection, and care. We don't feed for convenience—we feed to thrive.

When you nourish the whole household, you build a culture of lasting wellness.

CHAPTER 2

SNACKS

PACK YOUR POWER:
SNACKS & SMART LUNCHES

Midday nourishment that fuels energy, clarity, and real longevity

Your mid-day choices carry more weight than you think. They influence everything from your energy levels and focus to your digestion and mood. That's why I never leave the house without packing my own lunch, snacks, and supplements—whether I'm running errands, heading to an appointment, or traveling.

Why risk eating something that works against you?

We've all been there: grabbing something out of desperation, only to end up bloated, foggy, or regretful. It's not worth it. Convenience may seem tempting in the moment, but the cost to your body—your energy, your skin, your gut—is never worth the tradeoff.

Bringing your own food is about more than preference—it's about power. You control what goes in. You control how you feel.

ALWAYS PACK A LUNCH

Besides filtered water, I nearly always have a snack or small lunch on hand. This isn't a rigid routine—it's a lifestyle. One that supports vitality, digestion, and emotional stability throughout the day.

I've seen too many people eat out of desperation and spiral into discomfort: stomach upset, fatigue, brain fog. All avoidable. All unnecessary.

Packing your own food might seem minor, but there's quiet strength in consistency. In a world built on shortcuts, preparing your own nourishment is a quiet rebellion—one that pays off in clarity, balance, and true satisfaction.

WHAT'S IN MY BAG

What I bring varies depending on the season, my current goals, or how I'm feeling—but one thing never changes: I bring something.

My staples often include:

> Supplements: I take two 1000 mg MSM capsules with every meal. A Cayenne capsule for circulation and digestion. Occasionally a kelp supplement for iodine and trace minerals.
> Water: Always filtered or bottled—clean hydration matters.
> Snacks: Sliced veggies, boiled eggs, nuts (raw or dry roasted), pumpkin seeds, or pre-cooked meat cubes. Clean, simple, real.

Skip the Sandwich:
SMARTER, MEAT-BASED OPTIONS

I don't make sandwiches. And I rarely eat yeast-based breads. They simply don't serve me—they cause weight gain, sluggish digestion, and leave me feeling off. Even something as classic as a peanut butter and jelly sandwich triggers weight gain in our house—every time. It's not just the bread—it's the entire package of processed ingredients.

And deli meats? A hard no. Full of preservatives and nitrates, and are far from clean eating. If you're still leaning on deli meats, I encourage you to let them go. It might feel difficult at first, but what comes next is freedom—freedom from low-energy lunches and chemical-laden habits.

That's exactly how we started integrating cooked meat prep into our lives. I needed wholesome, ready-to-eat protein options that weren't loaded with chemicals. Now, I'll prep boneless, skinless chicken thighs ahead of time—cut them into cubes, store them, and they're ready to eat cold or warm. Turkey cutlets are another great option if you want variety.

One of our long-time staples is Mary's Organic Chicken. We've been buying it for years—every part of the bird. Even their chicken breast is juicy and never dry, and their wings are fantastic. When you find a truly high-quality meat, you don't get tired of it. It becomes an easy, go-to solution that tastes good and feels good.

CLEAN CRUNCH:
CELERY & CARROTS

Fiber, hydration, and real crunch—straight from the fridge

When it comes to natural fiber, hydration, and clean, energizing carbohydrates, raw vegetables like celery and carrots are my go-to. We've enjoyed them on and off for years—they're crisp, fresh, satisfying, and full of life. I like to keep them prepped and stored in the fridge for easy, grab-and-go fuel.

To keep carrots crisp, I buy them in bulk—usually a five-pound bag—and store them submerged in water. You can use a large glass jar or a big freezer bag. Just change the water every few days (at least once a week). When ready, peel, chop, and enjoy.

I use a similar method for celery. Buy a fresh bunch, trim the base and leafy tops, and place the stalks upright in a large glass jar with a few inches of water. Loosely cover it with a plastic bag and store it in the fridge. The celery stays vibrant and crunchy all week.

This same water method also works beautifully for fresh herbs like **parsley and cilantro,** which we use daily in our breakfast. I trim the stems and place the bunches in old jelly jars filled halfway with water. A loose plastic bag over the top (a bread bag works great) keeps them fresh for the week. It's a small trick that saves money, reduces waste, and keeps the greens we rely on ready to use.

These simple preps are easy, anti-aging habits that keep clean food within reach—every day.

SEEDS AND NUTS:
SMALL FOODS, BIG POWER

Fueling energy, brain health, and cellular protection with every handful

When it comes to building a youthful, resilient body, some of the most powerful foods are also the smallest. Seeds and nuts are compact power-houses—rich in clean fats, minerals, plant protein, and antioxidants that support brain clarity, joint health, smooth digestion, and lasting energy.

But not all nuts and seeds are created equal. For true anti-aging impact, the type you choose matters.

NUTS:
CLEAN ENERGY, BETTER BRAIN HEALTH

After years of testing, two nuts have proven themselves as true anti-aging allies in our routine:

▸ Macadamia nuts
▸ Walnuts

Macadamias are rich in monounsaturated fats—the same fats linked to heart health, insulin balance, and cognitive clarity. They're low in oxa-lates, making them gentler on the kidneys and ideal for daily digestion.

Walnuts are another powerhouse. Packed with plant-based omega-3 fatty acids, walnuts help protect brain cells, regulate inflammation, and support liver health. They also boost bone strength and feed the gut microbiome—critical pillars for aging well.

NUTS WE AVOID

Some nuts, while trendy, simply don't align with our goals:

 ‣ Almonds: Very high in oxalates, which can be burdensome to
   the kidneys and joints.
 ‣ Cashews: Delicious, but still moderate on the oxalate scale.

Choosing lower-oxalate options like macadamias and walnuts reduces internal stress while optimizing energy, digestion, and clarity.

Seeds:
NUTRIENT-DENSE, LOW-OXALATE SUPERFOODS

Our favorite seed by far is the pumpkin seed—a quiet but powerful superfood.

Pumpkin seeds are:

 ‣ Rich in magnesium, zinc, iron, and plant-based protein
 ‣ Low in oxalates
 ‣ Supportive of immune strength and blood sugar balance

We prefer roasting them ourselves:

 ‣ Use raw, unsalted pumpkin seeds
 ‣ Roast at 350°F for 20–30 minutes until golden and toasty

Store-bought versions often taste overcooked or flat. Roasting your own preserves the nutrients and enhances the flavor naturally.

> TIP FOR BEST RESULTS:
> Choose raw or lightly roasted nuts and seeds without added oils
> or flavorings.
> Portion intentionally—about a small handfull—so energy stays
> light, steady, and satisfying.

WHY SEEDS AND NUTS MATTER FOR ANTI-AGING

- Stabilize blood sugar and prevent energy crashes
- Fuel brain function with healthy fats and minerals
- Protect joints and tissues through anti-inflammatory compounds
- Support digestion without overwhelming the gut
- Deliver clean, lasting energy without the crash of processed snacks

CLEAN FUEL FOR BODY & BRAIN

A handful of carefully chosen nuts or seeds does more than curb hunger—it actively supports youthfulness. It supports digestion, fuels your brain, and delivers lasting nutrients without the crash or bloating of processed snack foods. By sticking to low-oxalate options like macadamias, walnuts, and pumpkin seeds, you're lightening your body's load while fueling it with what it truly needs.

Quick, portable, and deeply nourishing—these little foods pack big power. It's not just a snack. It's an anti-aging strategy in every bite.

HARD-BOILED EGGS:
THE ORIGINAL PROTEIN SNACK

Nature's portable fuel for strength, brain health, and youthful energy

Eggs are one of the most perfect foods ever created—a complete source of protein, packed with a powerful matrix of vitamins, minerals, and essential fats designed for optimal human nutrition.

For years, eggs carried an unfair reputation. Many people avoided them, fearing they would raise cholesterol levels. That caution steered countless individuals away from one of the most nourishing, bioavailable foods on earth—and into the arms of processed, chemically created "health" substitutes.

Quite the paradox.

If we simply chose the foods that God designed for us—rather than trusting lab-fabricated alternatives—we would spare our bodies the burden of detoxifying foreign substances disguised as fuel.

Real food builds strength naturally.

Fake food drains vitality silently.

NUTRITIONAL POWER IN EVERY EGG
Core Benefits:

▸ Complete protein for muscle maintenance
  Preserves lean tissue, supports metabolism, and strengthens recovery
▸ Choline for brain health
  Enhances memory, focus, and cognitive resilience
▸ Vitamin D and A for immune support and skin vitality
  Protects against cellular aging and strengthens defense systems
▸ Selenium and iodine for thyroid balance
  Boosts metabolic function and energy regulation
▸ Blood sugar stability
  Provides steady energy without crashes, supporting mental sharpness and physical endurance
▸ Digestive ease
  Naturally light, simple to digest, and free from additives or inflammatory triggers

Eggs offer a near-perfect food matrix—real nutrition that supports energy, hormone balance, tissue repair, mental sharpness, and digestive stability. They don't cause chaos in the body. They create order, resilience, and vibrant function from the inside out.

HOW WE PREPARE AND ENJOY HARD-BOILED EGGS
Every week, I make a batch of hard-boiled eggs as part of our regular food prep. They're clean, convenient, and completely unprocessed—true

grab-and-go nutrition. We don't rely on protein bars or "health snacks" packed with preservatives and seed oils. These are the original protein bars—crafted by nature, not a factory.

For lunches or snacks:

Slice the hard-boiled eggs in half

Spread with pasture-raised butter (our natural alternative to mayonnaise)

Season with Celtic sea salt, pepper, and sometimes a sprinkle of paprika, rosemary, coriander, or nutritional yeast for extra flavor and micronutrient boost

The result is a rich, satisfying, blood sugar-friendly food that energizes without inflaming the body.

HOW WE KEEP THEM FRESH ON THE GO

I keep it simple:

- Freeze water bottles ahead of time, pouring out about a quarter to allow expansion
- Use these frozen bottles as DIY ice packs for transporting lunches and snacks

Because I bring food with me almost everywhere I go, these ice packs get daily use—ensuring that real food stays fresh, cool, and ready when I need it.

Hard-boiled eggs aren't just a convenience. They're a conscious strategy: a pure, nutrient-dense food that protects youthfulness, sharpens the mind, supports strong digestion, and builds true, lasting vitality. In a world full of packaged shortcuts, real foods like eggs remain one of the simplest, smartest investments you can make in your health.

Homemade Yogurt:
CULTIVATING STRENGTH FROM THE INSIDE OUT

How building your microbiome supports energy,
mood, digestion, and youthful vitality

One of the most impactful additions to our health routine in recent years has been homemade probiotic yogurt—made fresh from carefully chosen strains designed to restore, fortify, and balance the gut microbiome.

The gut isn't just about digestion. It's your second brain, influencing your immunity, mood, hormonal balance, weight, cognitive function, and even your aging process. A strong, diverse gut microbiome is one of the most powerful anti-aging assets you can build—and daily probiotic foods are a key part of that strategy.

HOW OUR YOGURT JOURNEY BEGAN
We discovered this method after reading Super Gut by Dr. William Davis and watching demonstrations from Dr. Berg, among others. It looked simple—and it was.

We decided to invest in an Ultimate Probiotic Yogurt Maker, a small, specialized appliance made for long, low-temperature fermentation.

We now make Super Gut yogurt regularly at home, using a base of half-and-half (the recipe's suggested milk type for ideal consistency). We experimented with whole milk once, but it didn't culture properly and stayed watery. The half-and-half creates a rich, creamy, luxurious yogurt with the perfect texture—and an incredible flavor.

We were hooked from the first batch.

WHY THIS YOGURT IS DIFFERENT
This isn't commercial yogurt from the grocery store.

This is a 36-hour fermented probiotic powerhouse, designed to:
▸ Deliver billions of beneficial bacteria directly into the gut
▸ Strengthen gut barrier integrity

- ‣ Boost mood and emotional resilience
- ‣ Improve digestion and nutrient absorption
- ‣ Support immune function at the cellular level
- ‣ Reduce bloating, inflammation, and systemic aging triggers

It's truly a functional food—one that works at the deepest levels to support the systems that keep you strong, young, and mentally sharp.

HOW WE EAT IT

We split a small jar of our homemade yogurt each day, usually mid-day. Sometimes we add a spoonful of real fruit preserves for flavor—but even plain, the yogurt is smooth, creamy, and delicious.

It's also the perfect stand-in for sour cream. We spoon it over burritos, taco bowls, and even baked potatoes. The texture is thick, the flavor is tangy, and the live cultures make it a smarter, gut-friendly swap.

One important detail:

We always use wooden spoons for stirring and serving. Wood helps preserve the delicate structure of live cultures—and interestingly, it also helps raw honey dissolve better in our apple cider vinegar drinks. When working with living foods, natural tools make a real difference.

THE RESULTS WE'VE NOTICED

- ‣ Better digestion: More regularity, less bloating, stronger gut comfort
- ‣ Improved moods: A subtle but profound sense of greater emotional stability
- ‣ Stronger immune response: Feeling more resilient to environmental stresses

Adding homemade yogurt became a simple daily habit—but one that has yielded massive returns in how we feel, move, think, and live.

A vibrant gut creates a vibrant life.

If you're serious about sustaining youthful energy, clear thinking, smooth digestion, and emotional soundness, strengthening your microbiome isn't optional—it's essential. Homemade probiotic yogurt is one of the most efficient, natural ways to build that strength from the inside out.

Real yogurt. Real culture. Real nourishment.

Pork Rinds:
A SMART SNACK FOR NATURAL ENERGY AND HORMONE BALANCE

Choosing real fats to fuel metabolism, brain health, and youthful vitality

Sometimes the best snacks come from the most unlikely places.

Pork rinds have become a staple in our snack lineup—not as a guilty pleasure, but as a strategic source of clean, natural fats that support hormone health, energy balance, and metabolic strength.

WHY PORK RINDS WORK FOR HEALTH AND ANTI-AGING
Pork fat is a natural fat—rich in monounsaturated and saturated fats that the body uses to regulate hormones, build strong cell membranes, and maintain resilient skin and joints.

Unlike processed vegetable oils found in most commercial snacks, pork rinds contain no inflammatory seed oils, trans fats, or chemical emulsifiers.

Their benefits include:
- Supporting hormone synthesis (essential for metabolism, mood, skin, and mental clarity)
- Enhancing digestion and bile production (good fats stimulate healthy bile flow)
- Fueling the brain and stabilizing blood sugar without carbohydrate crashes
- Providing real, usable energy instead of a temporary sugar spike

Natural fats are a cornerstone of vibrant, youthful health—and pork rinds deliver them in a clean, simple, highly digestible form.

CHOOSING THE RIGHT PORK RINDS

Not all pork rinds are created equal.

We seek out brands with the simplest ingredient lists possible:

- Pork skins
- Salt
- Maybe a touch of clean seasoning (no MSG, no artificial flavors)

When you avoid processed chips loaded with seed oils, dyes, preservatives, and chemical flavorings, pork rinds become a genuinely smart alternative—especially compared to most snack foods on the market. *Key tip:* Always read the label. The shorter and more natural the ingredient list, the better.

WHY WE AVOID PROCESSED SNACK CHIPS

Even seemingly "simple" snacks like plain potato chips often hide dangers:

- Seed oils (like canola, soybean, corn) that are highly inflammatory
- Food dyes banned in other countries
- Residues from aluminum bags that can leach into food
- Preservatives that stress the liver and digestive system

Beyond ingredients, there's the unmistakable metallic aftertaste and sluggish feeling that follows eating most commercial chips. It's a reminder that these aren't real foods—they're industrial products disguised as snacks.

Every bite matters. Every snack is a choice between fueling your energy and youthfulness—or accelerating internal wear and tear.

PORK RINDS: THE SMART SWAP

Instead of reaching for processed chips, a handful of clean, minimally seasoned pork rinds offers:

- Real satisfaction
- Clean, usable energy
- Healthy fat intake that nourishes cells, hormones, and metabolism
- A crunchy, savory treat that fits into a truly anti-aging lifestyle

Choosing snacks intentionally keeps your body vibrant, clear, and resilient—long after the snack is gone.

BEVERAGES:
KEEP IT NATURAL, KEEP IT SIMPLE

Water is fundamental. It always has been. When you look around today, there's no shortage of beverage options—sodas, energy drinks, flavored waters, juices—but how many of them are truly natural? Not many. Companies love to splash the word "natural" across their packaging, but when you dig deeper, most of these drinks are anything but raw, pure, or unrefined.

Think back just two hundred years ago. What were people drinking? Mostly water. Sometimes vinegar mixed into water to help purify it. And of course, herbal teas—simple, ancient infusions made from real leaves, flowers, and roots. Not bottled concoctions loaded with processed additives, but true, clean plant extractions.

Today's beverage landscape is a far cry from that simplicity. Most options on the shelves are man-made chemical blends sweetened artificially or overloaded with sugars. Even so-called "100% juice" drinks are often little more than concentrated sugar fests. As kids, many of us drank Kool-Aid without giving it a second thought—colorful, sweet, and packed with artificial dyes. And now, the market is flooded with energy drinks, packed with synthetic stimulants, artificial colors, and who-knows-what else. I'm not even willing to try them. It's incredible how advertising shapes our desires for things we wouldn't naturally want.

Years ago, I started questioning it all.

Why the pressure to drink sodas?

Why the cultural expectation to consume sweetened carbonated beverages just to fit in?

Why is something natural often seen as strange, while chemical-laden drinks are celebrated?

I don't know if I have all the answers. But what I do know is this: choosing simplicity over trends is worth it. Every time you choose pure water, real herbal tea, or a naturally fermented beverage, you're giving your body a break—a gift, really. You're allowing your cells to focus on healing, hydration, and natural function instead of battling foreign chemical compounds.

Don't worry about stereotypes or what's considered "normal" by modern standards. Choose what feels right for your health and your energy. Natural beverages like clean water, real herbal teas, and traditionally brewed drinks like kombucha (made properly without excess sugars) support digestion, cellular repair, and mental clarity—without the hidden damage of artificial concoctions.

The simpler your beverages, the better your body will respond.

WATER:
THE TRUE FOUNDATION

Water remains the ultimate beverage for vitality. It hydrates your tissues, powers detoxification pathways, supports digestion, regulates temperature, and lubricates joints and skin. Every system in the body relies on proper hydration to work efficiently—and cellular dehydration is one of the silent accelerators of aging.

Our daily strategy:

▸ Start the day with structured hydration (apple cider vinegar water and a cranberry shot with lemon juice)
▸ Sip pure water throughout the day
▸ Carry a water bottle everywhere to stay proactive

HERBAL TEAS:
ANCIENT TOOLS FOR MODERN VITALITY

Herbal teas hydrate the body while delivering plant compounds that nourish, cleanse, and protect key systems like the liver, blood, digestion, and nervous system.

We prefer simple, straight herb teas—always organic when possible—not heavily processed blends or artificially flavored versions.

Our favorites include:

▸ Organic Green Tea (antioxidant powerhouse that protects cells and promotes metabolic health)
▸ Red Clover Tea (supports blood cleansing and healthy hormone balance)
▸ Nettle Tea (mineral-rich; strengthens blood, joints, skin, and hair)
▸ Yellow Dock Tea (stimulates gentle detoxification and supports liver and gut function)
▸ Fresh Ginger Tea (enhances digestion, improves circulation, reduces inflammation, and strengthens immune defenses)

These teas aren't just relaxing—they're active nourishment for the systems that sustain youthfulness, mental clarity, and internal resilience.

HOT LEMON WATER:
A SIMPLE DAILY DETOX

One of our favorite ways to refresh and reset is with hot lemon water. Simple yet powerful, it gently supports digestion, helps alkalize the body, boosts liver function, and naturally flushes out toxins—any time of day.

Hot lemon water also provides a light, natural dose of vitamin C and plant compounds that strengthen cellular health and connective tissue.

Benefits of hot lemon water include:

- ▸ Stimulating bile production for smoother digestion
- ▸ Gently cleansing the liver and kidneys
- ▸ Supporting healthy skin through internal hydration
- ▸ Boosting metabolism and improving nutrient absorption
- ▸ Providing antioxidant protection against daily oxidative stress

Adding hot lemon water to your day is one of the simplest, most effective strategies to keep your system moving, clear, and resilient.

BEVERAGES TO AVOID

Protect Your Body by Saying No to the Chemical Load

1. SODAS
Whether regular or diet, sodas are loaded with either high-fructose corn syrup or artificial sweeteners. Both promote inflammation, gut imbalance, and metabolic disruption. The carbonated acid load doesn't help either.

2. ENERGY DRINKS
Packed with synthetic caffeine, chemical stimulants, artificial colors, and mystery ingredients. These drinks may promise energy, but they tax the adrenal glands and burden the nervous system.

3. ARTIFICIALLY FLAVORED WATERS
Many "enhanced" waters contain fake sweeteners, dyes, preservatives, and chemical flavorings. Clean water shouldn't need a marketing campaign or a rainbow of colors.

4. COMMERCIAL FRUIT JUICES
Even 100% juices spike blood sugar and flood the body with more sugar than it was designed to process at once—without the natural fiber you'd get from eating the whole fruit.

5. PACKAGED "HEALTH" DRINKS

Protein shakes, sports drinks, and functional beverages often have long ingredient lists packed with synthetic vitamins, artificial flavors, emulsifiers, and gums. If it comes in a flashy package, it's worth questioning.

BOTTOM LINE:

Marketing makes these products sound healthy or cool.

Reality: they are stressors to your cells, your liver, and your longevity.

If you can't recognize or easily pronounce the ingredients, your body won't recognize them either. Stick to real, simple beverages that nourish—not burden—your system.

THE POWER OF NATURAL HYDRATION

Sticking to pure water, herbal teas, hot lemon water, and simple natural drinks doesn't just hydrate you—it cleanses, balances, and rebuilds the body every day.

It's a quiet discipline.

It's not flashy.

But the effects compound dramatically over time—supporting clearer skin, stronger digestion, sharper thinking, better hormone regulation, and smoother aging at the cellular level.

When you hydrate intentionally, you're not just drinking—you're fortifying your future health.

FUELING YOUTHFULNESS WITH EVERY CHOICE

Every bite, every sip, every small decision you make during the day either strengthens or stresses your body.

When you choose real foods—simple snacks made from natural ingredients, clean proteins, healthy fats, and pure hydration—you're doing more than avoiding processed traps.

You're actively building resilience into your cells, clarity into your mind, strength into your metabolism, and lightness into your energy.

Packing your own snacks, preparing your own lunches, and choosing beverages that truly nourish isn't about deprivation. It's about freedom— freedom from bloating, fatigue, brain fog, regret, and silent internal damage.

Every real food you choose becomes a small but powerful investment:
- Supporting smoother digestion
- Protecting hormone balance
- Preserving youthful skin, connective tissue, and joints
- Boosting mental sharpness and emotional stability
- Regulating blood sugar and metabolism naturally

In a culture that glorifies convenience over care, you're choosing to be different.

You're choosing to think long-term.

You're choosing to stay vibrant, sound-minded, and strong while the world around you quietly accelerates its own decline.

This is how real anti-aging happens:

One real food, one real choice, one real commitment at a time.

And the effects will show—not just in how you look, but in how you move, think, feel, and live.

"Real nourishment doesn't come with a barcode or a bright label. It comes from the earth."

CHAPTER 3

PREP IT UP

PRE-MAKING:
THE ART OF A WELL-RUN KITCHEN

Fueling your health by preparing with purpose

The best way to get the most out of cooking everything from scratch is through meal prep. Preparing as much as possible in advance allows me to utilize my time efficiently and stay ahead of the daily demands of real food living.

Cooking may take time—but for me, it's essential. It's a way of life, and it has become one of my favorite hobbies.

I'm constantly food planning:

- What needs to be defrosted?
- What's already prepped?
- What's next for dessert?
- What staples are running low?

There's always something to prepare—and every bit of preparation builds the foundation for the meals ahead.

Cooking is a way of life.

Or at least, it used to be.

Today, home cooking is becoming a lost art. Convenience culture has replaced the kitchen with drive-thrus and microwaveable boxes. Most food is either premade, processed, or handed over to someone else to prepare—usually with little concern for the quality of ingredients.

When you stop preparing your own food, you lose connection with what nourishes you. You surrender to chemicals, preservatives, and manufactured "foods"—a distorted version of what was once pure.

And make no mistake:

▸ These artificial foods don't help you look younger.
▸ They don't support vitality.
▸ They don't sustain clear thinking or balanced digestion.

They propel you toward dependency, inflammation, food addictions, and accelerated aging.

The disconnection goes deeper.

Today, many young people don't even know how to brew coffee.

Between coffee shop chains and Keurig pods, the idea of a traditional coffee pot has practically vanished from mainstream culture.

Even more striking, I recently spoke to a coworker who had never seen a cow in real life. The very animals that have sustained human life for thousands of years—the cow and the chicken—have been reduced to abstract products sold in neon-lit chains.

The population eats at McDonald's daily but has no direct connection to the reality of real food. (And as a side note, we can only hope they're still serving real meat.)

Preparing your own food isn't just a skill. It's a survival strategy.

It's a path back to vitality, youthfulness, and true nourishment. Cooking from scratch, planning ahead, and staying connected to your food isn't about being old-fashioned.

It's about taking full ownership of your health, your mind, and your future.

LEMON JUICE:
DAILY HEALTH BENEFITS AND EASY WEEKLY PREP

Simple strategies to detox, energize, and support youthful vitality

Fresh lemon juice is one of the easiest and most powerful tools you can add to your daily health routine.

It's simple, it's natural—and when used consistently, it can support digestion, boost detoxification, strengthen immune defenses, and even contribute to maintaining clearer, more youthful skin.

We use lemon juice both mornings and evenings as part of our core anti-aging strategy.

HEALTH BENEFITS OF FRESH LEMON JUICE

▸ *Stimulates digestion*
Activates bile production and digestive enzymes to help break down food efficiently
▸ *Alkalizes the body*
Despite its acidic taste, lemon juice leaves an alkaline residue in the body, supporting overall pH balance
▸ *Supports liver cleansing*
Enhances detoxification pathways and encourages the removal of waste and toxins
▸ *Provides antioxidants*
Delivers vitamin C and other natural compounds that protect cells and strengthen connective tissues
▸ *Boosts hydration*
Encourages better cellular hydration and mineral balance throughout the body

WEEKLY LEMON JUICE PREP

To make daily use simple, I press an entire bag of lemons at once using a citrus press. This produces about one to two cups of juice, which I store in a glass container in the refrigerator.

Fresh-pressed lemon juice keeps well for about 5–7 days, retaining its active nutrients and vibrant flavor. Having it ready removes the excuse of skipping—and makes staying consistent easy.

BONUS TIP:

Don't throw away the lemon rinds!

Toss a few into the garbage disposal to naturally cleanse the drain and freshen the kitchen with a burst of pure lemon scent.

FRESH GINGER:
A TIMELESS STAPLE FOR DIGESTION, IMMUNITY, AND VITALITY

One of nature's original tools for resilience and youthfulness

Fresh ginger root is a classic spice—timeless, powerful, and still one of the best tools we have for supporting digestion, calming inflammation, and strengthening natural immunity.

Its reputation stretches back through countless generations and cultures. From ancient herbal medicine to modern kitchens, ginger has remained a universal symbol of vitality and resilience.

HEALTH BENEFITS OF FRESH GINGER

- Enhances digestion
  Stimulates digestive enzymes and soothes the gastrointestinal tract
- Strengthens immune defenses
  Naturally antiviral, antimicrobial, and anti-inflammatory

- Reduces systemic inflammation
  Helps protect against aging processes driven by chronic internal inflammation
- Boosts circulation and metabolism
  Promotes healthy blood flow and natural detoxification pathways

HOW WE USE FRESH GINGER DAILY

Our favorite method is simple and powerful:

Fresh ginger tea, made right at home.

Here's how I prepare it:

- Peel and chop fresh ginger root into small cubes
- Portion the cubes into mini snack bags or containers for easy access
- In the evening, place a teaspoon to a tablespoon of ginger (depending on how spicy you like it) into a thermos
- Boil water and pour about 5–6 ounces per person over the ginger
- Seal the thermos and allow it to steep for at least an hour while we cook and eat dinner

By the time the meal is done, the tea is rich, warming, and ready to enjoy. Adding this simple ritual to your evenings quietly strengthens the systems that preserve youthfulness, resilience, and inner balance.

BEYOND SEED OILS: WHY WE MAKE OUR OWN TORTILLAS

Simple recipes that protect your health and expand your meal options

We used to buy a really good tortilla from Trader Joe's. And like many of our favorite clean products—it got discontinued. I tried so many other tortillas after that.

None of them compared. Most were loaded with poor-quality ingredients, especially seed oils, preservatives, and artificial conditioners. At that point, I decided everyone should be making their own tortillas. The difference in taste, texture, and health impact is incredible. Homemade tortillas are completely superior to anything you'll find on a store shelf.

OUR HOMEMADE TORTILLA ROUTINE
We use a simple recipe made with King Arthur flour and olive oil—clean, real, natural ingredients.

Here's how we batch them:
▸ Make three batches of dough, totaling about 36 tortillas
▸ Freeze them in sets of three (one for me, two for my husband)
▸ This creates twelve pre-portioned meals—enough to last for a couple months

Tortilla-making is definitely a team effort:
▸ I form the dough into golf ball-sized pieces
▸ My husband rolls them out
▸ I cook them in a paella pan, about 30 seconds per side

With one person rolling and one person flipping, the process moves quickly and efficiently.

WAYS WE USE HOMEMADE TORTILLAS
Homemade tortillas open up a wide variety of clean, satisfying dinner options:
▸ Simple side dish: Spread with butter and a sprinkle of salt
▸ Beef burritos: Using pre-cooked, seasoned ground beef
▸ Quesadillas: Filled with shredded homemade cheese and pre-prepped chicken

Because the tortillas are made from pure ingredients, they don't weigh you down or cause the bloating or inflammation you often feel from processed versions.

They're light, satisfying, and flexible enough to fit into a wide range of meals while still supporting digestion, energy, and overall vitality.

Real food, real ingredients, real energy.

Small shifts like making your own tortillas stack up to major gains in how you feel, move, and look every day.

ROASTED BEETS:
A TIMELESS FOOD FOR BLOOD HEALTH, DETOX, AND VITALITY

Simple prep, powerful nourishment

Through the years, we've switched up our appetizers many times. But roasted beets have stood the test of time—both in tradition and in proven health benefits.

Beets are loaded with a plethora of nutrients and phytochemical compounds that make them one of the most potent root vegetables you can add to your anti-aging strategy.

HEALTH BENEFITS OF ROASTED BEETS
- *Boost oxygenation and brain health*
  Natural nitrates in beets enhance blood flow, improving cognitive function and stamina.
- *Support red blood cell production*
  Their rich iron content helps regenerate healthy blood cells and support energy levels.
- *Stimulate liver function*
  Betaines found in beets aid detoxification and metabolic balance.
- *Strengthen overall immunity*
  Their dense nutrient profile fortifies the body against stress and environmental toxins.

Beets truly nourish from the inside out— fueling better circulation, sharper thinking , and deeper detoxification.

HOW WE PREP AND USE BEETS

Beets are definitely a dish best made with prep cooking in mind.

Here's how we prepare them:
- Preheat the oven to 425°F
- Place whole beets on a baking sheet
- Drizzle lightly with olive oil, Celtic sea salt, and black pepper
- Cover tightly with aluminum foil
- Bake for about one hour, depending on beet size

After roasting:
- Peel the skins off easily by hand (or using a paper towel)
- Slice into ¼-inch rounds

Like all our prep-cooked dishes, I portion the slices into small sandwich bags and freeze them.

Each bag contains just a few slices—perfect for a daily or occasional appetizer.

The night before, simply transfer a bag to the refrigerator to thaw gently.

Serving Tip: Sprinkle with a touch of Celtic sea salt for a simple, nourishing appetizer packed with flavor and nutrients.

OXALATE CAUTION

Beets are on the higher side for oxalates, which are natural compounds that can contribute to mineral buildup if consumed in excess. If you're following a low-oxalate diet or managing kidney health, it's best to enjoy beets occasionally rather than daily.

Real root. Real blood flow. Real detox.

BONE BROTH:
A TIMELESS STRATEGY FOR GUT, JOINTS, AND VITALITY

Rebuilding from the inside out, one cup at a time

Many years ago, we started making homemade bone broth—and it's become a cornerstone of our nutrition strategy.

Bone broth is a timeless tradition across many cultures.

WHY BONE BROTH MATTERS FOR HEALTH AND YOUTHFULNESS

- *Strengthens joints and connective tissues*
  Rich in collagen, gelatin, and natural compounds that protect flexibility and mobility
- *Repairs and protects the gut lining*
  Nourishes intestinal health, supporting digestion and stronger immunity
- *Boosts bone strength naturally*
  Supplies bioavailable calcium, magnesium, and phosphorus
- *Improves skin elasticity and hydration*
  Collagen supports smoother, firmer skin and slows visible signs of aging
- *Supports faster recovery and tissue repair*
  Supplies amino acids crucial for healing and energy renewal
- *Enhances hair, nails, and dental health*
  Strengthens keratin and mineral balance across the body

HOW WE MAKE BONE BROTH

We invested in a six-gallon stock pot to make large batches, ensuring we always have plenty on hand.

Our typical recipe uses:

- 14–15 pounds of chicken parts (primarily chicken feet and necks, for maximum collagen and gelatin content)
- Celery, carrots, fresh parsley
- Celtic sea salt and black pepper
- Apple cider vinegar (to help extract minerals and gelatin from the bones)

The result is a richly gelatinous broth, loaded with the building blocks the body needs to repair tissues, protect joints, and support digestive and immune health. *(The recipe is in the back of the book or you can watch the demo on my YouTube channel).*

PORTIONING AND STORAGE

After simmering for hours and cooling slightly, we strain the broth and portion it into plastic restaurant-style containers.

Each batch yields an average of forty-five servings. We freeze the servings immediately for freshness and convenience. When ready to enjoy, we simply heat a portion in a small cast iron saucepan. My husband and I typically split one serving together for a daily boost of digestible, bioavailable nutrition.

BONE BROTH FOR DOGS

Our dogs benefit from bone broth too! They get a couple spoonfuls alongside their dinner to help support their joints, coat, and agility.

Important Tip:

If you're making broth to share with pets, omit garlic and onions, which are toxic to dogs. We made that adjustment after learning from our earliest batches!

Bone broth isn't just comfort food—it's a timeless daily strategy that nourishes the body, preserves youthfulness, and fortifies resilience from the inside out.

Noodles:
FAST, FLEXIBLE, AND MEAL-PREP FRIENDLY

Simple fuel for real life on the go

Time and time again, we've found ourselves needing clean, satisfying meals ready to go. One of the best recent innovations in our kitchen is prep-cooked noodles.

HOW WE PREP NOODLES
The process is simple and efficient:
- Boil a bag of dried noodles in a pasta pot
- Drain, cool, and divide the noodles into eight single-serving portions
- Place each portion into a plastic sandwich bag
- Store all the small bags inside a gallon freezer bag and freeze

Now we always have perfectly portioned, ready-to-use noodles available whenever we need a fast meal.

NOODLE MEAL COMBINATIONS
You can combine noodles with almost any pre-cooked meat for a balanced, nourishing meal:
- Ground beef or ground lamb
- Cubed chicken or pork

Simple assembly:
- Place a bag of noodles and some pre-cooked meat into a pan with a lid or a Crockpot
- Let it warm together
- Add a simple sauce, seasoning, or condiment at the end if desired

Real food, fast, without sacrificing quality, digestion, or energy.

Small strategies like these make the difference between grabbing something processed—and staying on the path toward vitality and resilience.

CORN SPOON BREAD:
HONORING TRADITION WITH SMART MEAL PREP

A timeless food, made simple for modern life

Corn has been a constant staple across civilizations for centuries.

A timeless food source, rich with history, nourishment, and comfort—it's something nearly everyone recognizes and loves.

Years ago, I was searching for a cornbread recipe for Thanksgiving. I found an old Native American cookbook with a simple corn recipe. I thought it would be traditional cornbread—but it turned out to be closer to a quiche-like texture, with a surprising lightness from the eggs. Soft, rich, and deeply satisfying.

HOW WE MAKE AND STORE IT
I bake this corn dish in a 9x13-inch cake pan.

Once cooled, I cut it into eight squares, and freeze each piece individually in sandwich bags. This makes it easy to grab exactly what we need without waste. *(The full recipe is in the recipe section at the back.)*

To reheat:
- Preheat the oven to 300°F
- Bake the frozen piece for 30–40 minutes
- By the time I get home from work and settle in, it's warmed perfectly—without any rush or hassle

Top it with a little butter and honey for a beautiful, simple finish. Without a doubt, this is one of the best fast foods. All natural, handmade, nourishing—and far superior to anything in a drive-thru window.

Small strategies like these make the difference between grabbing something processed—and staying on the path toward vitality and resilience.

BUTTER COOKIES:
THE PERFECT CLEAN TREAT

Simple ingredients, real satisfaction

You can never go wrong with a classic shortbread cookie.

I like to call them butter cookies—because that's exactly what they are: clean, simple, rich, and real.

These cookies are an exemplary baked good.

- Great for lunch
- Perfect after dinner with tea
- Simple enough to fit into any real-food lifestyle without sabotage

THE BEAUTY OF A MINIMAL INGREDIENT LIST

One of the best things about these cookies is how few ingredients they require.

Just five—and they're all pure and straightforward:

- Butter (pasture-raised, high-quality)
- Flour (unbleached, organic)
- Sugar (just half a cup, to keep it lightly sweet)
- Vanilla (always real, never imitation)
- Pecans (raw or dry roasted—never oil-roasted)

The fewer the ingredients, the better the digestibility, energy stability, and satisfaction.

Simple, no-nonsense nourishment—even in a cookie.

WHY CLEAN TREATS MATTER
Small choices, lasting impact
  - *Better digestion*
    Simple ingredients are easier for the body to break down and
    assimilate
  - *No inflammatory oils*
    Avoid hidden seed oils that trigger inflammation, gut issues, and
    aging processes
  - *Stable blood sugar*
    Less sugar means fewer energy crashes and better hormonal
    balance
  - *Real satisfaction*
    Nutrient-dense treats satisfy cravings without leaving you feel-
    ing bloated or sluggish
  - *Support for youthful vitality*
    Even desserts can strengthen—not sabotage—your journey
    toward lasting health

HOW WE MAKE AND STORE THEM
I make two batches at once, then flash freeze them after baking.
   Pro tip:
You can eat these cookies almost straight from the freezer—they
defrost incredibly fast and retain a perfect texture.

INGREDIENT NOTES
  - Flour:
    I love Arrowhead Mills organic flour—light, unbleached, and
    perfect for delicate pastries.
  - Nuts:
    Always choose raw or dry roasted pecans.
    If nuts are roasted with oils, you're likely getting exposed to
    rancid seed oils—highly inflammatory and counterproductive to
    a health-focused lifestyle.

Keeping even your treats clean makes a real difference in how your body feels and responds long-term.

(You'll find the cookie recipe tucked in the recipes section at the back.)

Real food isn't about deprivation—it's about upgrading even your desserts to nourish, satisfy, and support your energy and vitality.

REAL DESSERTS:
SATISFYING THE SWEET TOOTH WITHOUT SABOTAGING HEALTH

Pure ingredients, real satisfaction, lasting vitality

Just because we're committed to vibrant health doesn't mean we're skipping dessert.

Quite the opposite. I fully appreciate a sterling confection to beautifully culminate a nourishing meal.

But here's the difference:

‣ It must be made from scratch
‣ It must use pure, real ingredients
‣ It must support, not sabotage, the body's energy, digestion, and vitality

I maintain a broad array of homemade desserts in our house—always prepared ahead to avoid the classic "slippery slope" into commercial, processed, artificial options that so many people surrender to when sugar cravings hit.

LEMON TARTS:
A FRESH, TANGY STAPLE

One of our favorite desserts is the homemade lemon tart.

- ▸ I make the crusts from scratch, ensuring pure ingredients and light texture.
- ▸ We bake three pies at a time for efficiency.
- ▸ My husband helps prepare the custard filling.

Batch prepping desserts together isn't just about practicality—it's an investment in health, connection, and community. Cooking side by side strengthens relationships just as much as it strengthens the body.

Freezer Tip:

Lemon tarts freeze beautifully.

They come out tasting just as fresh as the day they were made.

PECAN PIE:
SWEETNESS WITHOUT COMPROMISE

Another staple in our kitchen is homemade pecan pie, enjoyed with a scoop of Straus pasture-raised vanilla ice cream.

- ▸ We make three pies at a time, cut into six slices each, and freeze individually.
- ▸ Unlike many commercial recipes, our version uses brown sugar and butter—no corn syrup, no oils.
- ▸ Vital Farms pasture-raised eggs give it superior flavor and nutrient density.

Again, freezing keeps the pies perfectly fresh without the need for the preservatives and chemicals found in store-bought versions.

BUTTER CAKE:
A BITE OF REAL FLAVOR

One more dessert I always have on hand is a rich, simple butter cake, baked in a Bundt pan.

- ‣ Cut into 18–20 individual servings
- ‣ Light, flavorful, and fully satisfying without being heavy or overwhelming

We're not trying to be full—we're aiming for a few bites of real satisfaction. When you enjoy a properly prepared, nutrient-dense dessert, you're not "missing out" at all.

You're avoiding the crash, the inflammation, the regret—and preserving the vitality, digestion, and mental clarity that processed foods steal away.

Healthy living isn't about deprivation—it's about upgrading every bite to nourish body, mind, and spirit.

Even dessert can be part of your daily anti-aging, vitality-supporting lifestyle when made with intention and pure ingredients.

DOG MEAL PREP:
REAL FOOD FOR LONGEVITY AND VITALITY

Simple homemade strategies to keep your pets thriving

Our dogs are part of the family—and just like us, they deserve real, nourishing food to support strong bodies, sharp minds, and long, vibrant lives.

We don't rely on commercial dog food as their main source of nutrition. Kibble is reserved as a light snack only. For dinner, we prepare a variety of clean, home-cooked foods—rich in natural proteins, vegetables, and minerals—made with the same care and intention we bring to our own meals.

CHICKEN AND TURKEY PREP

The main protein for our dogs' dinners is chicken thighs.

Here's how we prepare it:
- Purchase about 15 pounds of chicken thighs
- Bake at 350°F for 50 minutes on baking sheets
- Once cooled, chop into 1-inch pieces
- Divide into daily serving bags (sandwich-sized zip bags) and freeze

Each day, we simply move one bag from the freezer to the fridge. Always fresh. Always simple.

So much better than dry, processed dog food.

For variety, we also use ground turkey:
- Bake 4 pounds of ground turkey at 350°F (right on a baking sheet)
- Once cooked, chop and divide into daily portions
- Freeze just like the chicken

Rotating proteins helps ensure a broader spectrum of nutrients and keeps mealtimes exciting for them.

RICE PREP

We make 1 cup of rice in a rice cooker to serve alongside their protein. The rice is stored in a glass container in the refrigerator and lasts a week. At dinner, we boil water and splash a little over their meal to moisten the rice and gently warm the food without overheating it.

VEGETABLE PREP

Fresh vegetables are an essential part of our dogs' dinners.

We pre-chop an assortment and keep them ready in sandwich bags in the fridge for quick access.

Vegetables we regularly use include:
- Red and green cabbage
- Green or yellow summer squash

These add fiber, vitamins, minerals, and important plant compounds to support digestion, detoxification, and cellular health.

BUTTERNUT SQUASH PREP

Butternut squash is another powerful addition—rich in potassium, fiber, and antioxidants.

Here's how we prepare it:
- Cut the squash in half
- Bake at 375°F for 30 minutes
- Slice into five pieces per half
- Freeze daily portions in sandwich bags

Every couple days, the dogs get about a one-inch cube of squash. It's the perfect amount for small dogs—enough to deliver nutrients without upsetting digestion.

PUMPKIN SEEDS FOR ADDED NUTRITION

Pumpkin seeds are an easy superfood for dogs—packed with fiber, healthy fats, and minerals.

After roasting seeds for ourselves, I grind a batch for the dogs using a mortar and pestle.

I store the ground seeds in a glass container and give one teaspoon daily with their dinner.

REAL FOOD. REAL HEALTH

Feeding our dogs fresh, real food isn't complicated—it just takes a little planning.

In return, they stay vibrant, energetic, sharp-minded, and visibly healthy. Just like humans, animals thrive when given the natural nutrition they were designed for.

CHAPTER 4

APPETIZERS AND DINNER

WHY DINNER PREPARES YOU FOR TOMORROW'S ENERGY AND LONGEVITY

My husband always jokes that it takes "a hundred steps to make dinner."

He might be right.

I think he started helping me cook 25 years ago simply because he wanted to eat.

Between chopping this, slicing that, and my usual insistence that "I'm not eating unless there are fresh vegetables," dinner prep can definitely be a process—but it's worth every step.

In our home, my husband handles all the meat:

- He cooks the eggs for breakfast
- He prepares the main proteins for dinner

I'm the prep cook—washing, chopping, seasoning, and assembling all the fruits and vegetables. Together, we make 99% of our meals from scratch.

Why?

Because real food is the foundation of health, vitality, and a sound mind. Non-processed is the secret.

WHY WE CHOOSE REAL FOOD

People are often surprised when I describe our meals—eggs, bacon, burgers, pancakes—and respond with comments like:

"Oh, you just don't care what you eat."

"You're really letting yourself go."

But the truth is the opposite. We eat incredibly well.

We eat food that tastes amazing, that's full of healthy fats and real flavor—and we feel vibrant doing it.

The secret is simple:

WE MAKE IT ALL OURSELVES.

We use mostly organic ingredients when possible, but more importantly, we avoid processed foods. Processing doesn't just add preservatives—it destroys the integrity of the food itself.

- ‣ Nutrients degrade.
- ‣ Textures change.
- ‣ Chemicals enter the picture.

And don't even get me started on GMOs.

When a food is genetically modified, its chemical structure shifts beyond what our digestive systems were designed to recognize.

The human body was made for whole foods—not lab-fabricated products sprayed with pesticides and cloaked in preservatives.

THE POWER OF READING LABELS

Making everything from scratch might not be perfect. Nothing is. But it's one of the most powerful choices you can make to retain control over your health, digestion, and longevity.

When we cook, we use:

- ‣ Single, real ingredients that don't require a label—or, if they do, list only one pure item.
- ‣ If something has multiple ingredients, we read every single word.

We look for real food—not chemicals, fillers, or emulsifiers. Try finding a hot sauce without xanthan gum. It's not easy.

And if a chemical is listed, imagine how many other additives were included in tiny amounts too small to legally require a mention. Finding trustworthy brands matters.

Your health is worth the extra step.

Clean Food. Clear Mind. Lasting Youth.

Every ingredient you skip or select today shapes how you feel, look, and age tomorrow.

WHY MAKING DINNER MATTERS

Small efforts, powerful rewards

▸ *Supports better digestion*
Real foods are easier to break down and nourish the gut lining naturally
▸ *Improves nutrient density*
Home-cooked meals maximize vitamins, minerals, and absorption
▸ *Stabilizes energy and blood sugar*
Balanced meals without hidden sugars or additives sustain vitality throughout the evening and overnight
▸ *Strengthens hormonal balance*
Natural fats and whole foods support thyroid, adrenal, and metabolic function
▸ *Enhances sleep quality*
Properly fueled bodies experience deeper, more restorative sleep—essential for youthfulness and cognitive clarity
▸ *Builds long-term resilience*
Every clean dinner strengthens the body's ability to repair, rebuild, and protect itself against aging and stress

MAGNESIUM LEMON DRINK:
A SIMPLE PRE-DINNER BOOST

To go along with dinner, I like to prepare a simple magnesium drink.

Here's what I use:

- ▸ Powdered magnesium citrate (preferred over capsules for better absorption)
- ▸ Fresh lemon juice (about 1–2 tablespoons)

I mix the magnesium powder with water until it fully dissolves, then stir in the lemon juice.

The lemon provides natural acidity to enhance digestion and prepare the body for the upcoming meal.

Even the dogs have their own version of this "dinner booster"—just in a much smaller amount.

Dog Prep Tip:

- ▸ I use a set of tiny "dot" and "smidge" measuring spoons for their supplements.
- ▸ I mix a tiny amount of magnesium powder into about two tablespoons of water and pour it into their dinner bowls (usually chicken and rice).
- ▸ For the dogs, I skip the lemon juice and simply offer the mineral boost alone.

> ### MAGNESIUM LEMON DRINK
>
> - 1 teaspoon magnesium citrate
> - 6 ounces water
>
> Stir till magnesium dissolves clear
> Add 1-2 tablespoon lemon juice

> ### DOG MAGNESIUM
>
> - 1-2 tablespoon water
> - 1 smidge spoon magnesium citrate
>
> Swirl in glass till dissolved (20 seconds)

APPETIZERS

APPETIZERS WITH PURPOSE:
SIMPLE STARTS THAT NOURISH

Sometimes the best ways to nourish your body are also the simplest. Adding health-boosting vegetables, fruits, and herbs to your meals doesn't have to involve elaborate recipes. In fact, some of the most effective foods for skin, digestion, brain health, and hormone support are the easiest to prepare. A few well-chosen ingredients can become a consistent part of your daily rhythm—and bring noticeable results with very little effort.

CUCUMBERS:
COOLING, CLEANSING, AND BRAIN-SUPPORTIVE

Adding vegetables to your diet can be as easy as slicing a cucumber. These refreshing green staples are packed with fiber, hydration, and health-promoting phytonutrients. They support healthy skin, reduce inflammation, and provide vitamin K, which plays a role in cognitive function. Cucumbers also contain flavonoids that may help protect the brain from oxalate-related damage.

They make a great appetizer, and even our dogs enjoy them as a light, hydrating treat. Fresh, clean, and easy—cucumbers are a daily go-to for us.

AVOCADO SALAD:
FIBER, FATS, AND ANTIOXIDANTS

Avocados are one of the most nutrient-dense fruits you can eat. They're loaded with healthy fats, antioxidants, and vitamins, including more potassium than a banana. Their carotenoids help prevent oxidative stress, and their fiber content supports digestion and blood sugar balance.

One of our favorite starters is a simple avocado salad. I chop one avocado, a tomato, and some cucumber, then add one tablespoon each of apple cider vinegar and organic extra virgin olive oil per person. Add a pinch of salt and pepper, mix well, and serve chilled. It's incredibly refreshing and energizing.

TORTILLA CHIPS WITH BUTTER
AND A ROSEMARY TWIST

This one may sound a little unusual—but sometimes unconventional ideas become everyday favorites. One day I was craving butter and thought: people butter corn and popcorn, so why not corn chips? I dipped a tortilla chip in butter and loved it. Eventually my husband tried it too, and now it's a staple snack for us.

Yes, tortilla chips are fried in seed oils, and yes, they make our "more than one ingredient" list—but the brand we buy from Trader Joe's has a relatively clean label. Moderation is key. A single bag lasts us about a week.

To get even more benefit from this snack, I've started sprinkling rosemary on the buttered chips. Rosemary has become a daily addition to my routine because of its hormone-balancing and brain-boosting properties. It stimulates circulation, improves skin health, protects against UV damage, and has antimicrobial and anti-inflammatory effects. It also supports hormone regulation in both men and women. I used to experience frequent night sweats, but since adding rosemary daily, they've completely disappeared.

EASY CHOICES, LASTING BENEFITS
These foods may seem simple, but they offer meaningful support for your skin, mind, digestion, and hormones. You don't have to overhaul your diet or spend hours in the kitchen to start feeling better—just focus

on high-impact ingredients you can easily work into your daily habits. Whether it's cucumbers with dinner, an avocado salad mid day, or a rosemary-sprinkled chip, small choices can lead to big improvements. Wellness doesn't have to be complicated—it just has to be intentional.

MAIN MEALS

Meats:
REAL FOOD, REAL FLAVOR

Meat has long been a staple in our household, but how we prepare and source it has evolved over the years. Like most Americans, we started out making simple burgers from store-bought meat. But with time—and a lot of trial and error—we've learned the difference that quality sourcing, preparation, and thoughtful ingredients can make. From pasture-raised beef to carefully chosen spices and sauces, our meals are built around real, recognizable food. This section highlights some of our favorite ways to enjoy meats while minimizing additives and maximizing flavor, nutrition, and satisfaction.

BETTER BURGERS START WITH BETTER BEEF
We've made burgers for years, but the quality of the meat makes all the difference. We used to buy organic ground beef from the store, but freezing it ruined the texture. Eventually, we started buying grass-fed beef through local food co-ops. If you haven't tried it, I highly recommend exploring co-ops in your area. Pasture-raised beef is ideal, but grass-fed is a solid second choice. And if that's unavailable, even store-bought beef is better than any over-processed product.

The difference in flavor and integrity with co-op beef is significant—and it freezes beautifully without altering taste or texture. I tested several co-ops before finding our favorite, and I suggest trying a few to see which suits your preference best.

Cooking Technique:
SKIP THE GRILL, KEEP THE JUICE

While we used to barbecue our burgers, we discovered a better method when making sliders for the Super Bowl one year. Inspired by cast iron skillet recipes, we started cooking our burgers in a Dutch oven. This method locks in the juices and creates a moist, flavorful patty that beats anything off the grill—especially since grilling causes valuable fats to drip away. Since healthy fats support the brain, skin, and overall vitality, we make it a point to keep them in the dish, not in the flames.

We shape our patties by hand using just beef, salt, and pepper. Cook them for 4–5 minutes per side in a preheated Dutch oven. Let them rest a few minutes after cooking to reabsorb the juices and reach their peak texture and flavor.

BUN-FREE AND BETTER THAN EVER
We stopped using hamburger buns years ago when we realized we couldn't find one we liked. Most are ultra-processed and full of mystery ingredients. Once we eliminated them, the burgers actually tasted better. We serve them bunless on a warmed plate, layered with organic ketchup, chopped garlic, Jalapeños, Fresno peppers, and Serrano peppers. Then we top the patties with real cheddar cheese and place them in the oven briefly to melt. The result is a clean, flavorful, nutrient-rich dish—no bread necessary.

Wings and Pizza:
A SMARTER PAIRING

Chicken wings are a regular dinner in our home. We prep and freeze them ourselves, then bake the defrosted wings at 375°F for 25 minutes after tossing them in olive oil and whatever spice blend we're craving. Cayenne, Habanero, and Thai chili powder are a few of our favorite heat options—clean, simple, and bold.

We often pair the wings with something that might surprise you: Trader Joe's organic cheese pizza. I know frozen pizza might sound like an unhealthy choice, but it's better to satisfy a craving with something you've chosen intentionally, rather than grabbing takeout made with mystery oils and questionable ingredients. When you control what comes through your door, you're already ahead.

We eat foods that are, in themselves, the ingredient. One item. One name. That's our rule. If something has a label, it better be short—and it better be worth it.

There are fewer than ten products in our kitchen with an actual ingredient list. And even then, it's a short one. These are our carefully chosen exceptions:

- Ketchup (organic, no corn syrup)
- Tortilla chips (organic corn, oil, salt)
- Butter croissants (butter, flour, salt—no seed oils)
- Cheese pizza (clean sauce, mozzarella, olive oil crust)
- Fruit preserves (just fruit and sugar)
- Straus vanilla ice cream (cream, milk, sugar, vanilla)
- Hot sauce (peppers, vinegar, salt—no additives)
- Coconut aminos (coconut sap and salt)

We don't aim for perfection, but we do aim for clarity. If we can't pronounce it, we don't buy it. If it has more than five ingredients, it probably doesn't make the cut.

NACHO NIGHT:
HEAT, FLAVOR, AND CLEAN INGREDIENTS

Another go-to is Nacho Night. We brown ground beef and mix in a homemade spice blend. For toppings, we go heavy on flavor and heat—Jalapeños, Fresno, and Serrano peppers, chopped garlic, and a generous amount of shredded cheddar and habanero jack cheeses.

We shred our own cheese to avoid the anti-caking agents and fillers found in store-bought shredded blends. We finish it all with a clean hot sauce—ideally with a short ingredient list and no thickeners like xanthan gum. Our favorite right now is from Generalshotsauce.com, which offers a grenade-shaped bottle and a range of bold, flavorful options.

BAKED FRENCH FRIES:
A HEALTHIER TAKE ON A CLASSIC

Homemade French fries are the perfect side for burgers—and when you bake them instead of deep frying, they become a much healthier option. We make ours in the oven, and the result is surprisingly satisfying with a crisp texture and clean flavor.

I use a French fry press, which quickly cuts potatoes into even, classic fry shapes. After pressing, I soak the potato slices in a bowl of water for a few minutes to draw out excess starch. Then I pat them dry with a paper towel, toss them in olive oil, and sprinkle with salt.

Bake them on a cookie sheet at 425°F for about 40 minutes. The result is golden, crisp, and full of flavor—without the heaviness of frying. Honestly, I'm surprised this isn't the go-to method for more people. The texture and taste speak for themselves.

SPICES THAT MATTER:
WHY WE SWITCHED TO CLEANER SPICES

When you're preparing meals from scratch, every ingredient matters—right down to your spice rack.

Spices are small but mighty. They can elevate a dish, support digestion, and even provide powerful antioxidants. But here's what most people don't realize: many store-bought spices contain hidden fillers, flow agents, or additives that aren't listed on the label. These invisible extras can interfere with how your body absorbs other nutrients—and in some cases, they can cause surprising reactions.

That's why we made a change.

We learned firsthand how additives in spice blends can interfere with other ingredients. One brand of garlic powder left us unable to enjoy salt—something in the anti-clumping agent seemed to throw off how our bodies processed minerals. Once we stopped using that garlic, we could enjoy Celtic sea salt again with no issues.

That led us to search for a higher-quality spice company. We found SpicesInc.com, which sells pure, filler-free dried spices. Yes, some of their spices may clump a little more—but we'll take that over added flow agents any day. The flavors are stronger, the textures are cleaner, and our food tastes better as a result.

THE REAL DIFFERENCE REAL FOOD MAKES

When you start choosing real meat, clean spices, and unprocessed ingredients, something shifts—not just in the flavor of your meals, but in how you feel day to day. Meals become energizing instead of draining. You stay full longer, think more clearly, and feel more balanced overall. It's not about being gourmet—it's about returning to simple, nutrient-dense food that works with your body instead of against it. Real food, thoughtfully prepared, is one of the best investments you can make in your vitality.

Choose spices that are as real as the rest of your food. It's a small shift that makes a powerful difference.

MEALS TO GO:

Taking Real Food with You

HEALTHY FOOD WHEREVER YOU ARE

Eating clean, nourishing meals doesn't have to stop just because you're away from home. Whether your schedule is unpredictable or you're simply on the go, planning ahead makes it possible to enjoy home-cooked food anywhere. We've prepared many of our dinners to-go over the years, and it's been the key to avoiding processed food or the temptation of eating out. There's no need for excuses—just preparation and a few smart tools.

If eating meals at home isn't an option, here's some suggestions on taking delicious healthy foods with you. We've prepared many of our dinners to take to-go when our schedules fluctuated. There's no excuses for why you have to eat out or choose processed foods.

GRAB-AND-GO CHICKEN AND COLESLAW

One of our favorite travel-friendly meals is chicken legs and coleslaw. After baking a batch of chicken, I separate the legs into individual snack bags, then place them all in a large freezer Ziplock. This makes it easy to grab just what you need. They can be eaten warm or cold—both ways are delicious.

The coleslaw is best made the day before to give it time to chill and develop flavor. I keep it clean and simple with vinegar and oil—no mayonnaise. Most store-bought mayo is made with inflammatory seed oils, so we skip it entirely. This dinner is low-carb, refreshing, and satisfying. If you want to round it out, add a buttered croissant or a slice of homemade sourdough.

THE MINI CROCK POT SOLUTION

We found a small, single-serving crock pot designed for travel—it's been a game-changer. Just plug it in an hour before lunch, and your meal is warm and ready with zero chance of overcooking. It's perfect for simple, hearty meals like a protein paired with rice or noodles.

MEAL IDEAS WITH GROUND MEATS AND RICE

Ground meats are quick and easy to prepare. One go-to combo is ground beef and rice. Brown the beef in a pan, cook rice in a stainless steel rice cooker, and layer them in the mini crock pot. You can add frozen broccoli for extra nutrients—it heats up beautifully. A splash of coconut aminos finishes it off with a satisfying umami flavor.

Ground lamb is another great option. Cook it simply with salt and pepper. For larger other cuts of meat, cube steak, pork or chicken into small pieces so they cook quickly on the stovetop and fit easily into the to-go container.

Rice is a prefect pairing for any of these meats. I use a rice cooker that has a stainless steel insert instead of the toxic nonstick variety. You can even substitute the rice with the premade noodles. I prep cooked the noodles. Then portion into individual serving sizes. Store in individual ready to eat bags in the freezer.

These are a few simple variations to make great meals. I will say the better the quality of the meat you buy, the more you won't want to add to much else to it. With the cost of fast food these days, home cooking isn't more expensive. A pound of organic grass fed ground beef averages around eight to ten dollars a pound. Rice and noodles are less than a dollar.

Real health isn't about perfect circumstances—it's about building the habits and systems that keep you strong, no matter where life takes you.

DESSERTS:
SWEETNESS THAT SUPPORTS HEALTH AND VITALITY

Homemade treats with real ingredients and real benefits

WHY WE STILL EAT DESSERT
When you're trying to stay healthy, it might seem like dessert has to disappear—but it doesn't. In our home, we enjoy desserts regularly. The key is simple: they must be homemade and built with real, unprocessed ingredients.
- Less sugar
- Real fats like butter or coconut oil
- No condensed milk, no seed oils, no artificial additives

I usually make homemade buttermilk for recipes by adding one tablespoon of apple cider vinegar to a cup of milk. Let it sit for 5–10 minutes, and you have a more digestible, lightly fermented milk that lifts the texture and nutritional quality of any cake or pastry.

COCONUT OIL CAKES:
A SURPRISING DISCOVERY

Years ago, we baked almost everything with coconut oil.

At that time, it was the trend—and it's still a worthy one.

The Bundt cakes we made using coconut oil were spectacular, and surprisingly, the more we ate, the slimmer our body composition became. It sounds counterintuitive—dessert every night and better weight control—but the high-quality fats in coconut oil helped support metabolism, regulate digestion, and keep cravings balanced.

Good fats have a real-life impact: they help lower cortisol, support the brain, and contribute to deep, restorative sleep. Although we eventually transitioned to baking with butter more than the coconut oil, the core principle remains:

Healthy fats are foundational for health, vitality, and youthful resilience.

PECAN SANDIES:
SIMPLICITY AND SATISFACTION

Another dessert we still enjoy is homemade butter cookies—what many know as pecan sandies.

- Simple, real ingredients: flour, butter, sugar, pecans.
- Tiny cookies—only about two inches across—enjoyed in moderation.

We don't eat desserts to feel "full."

We eat to feel satisfied, uplifted, and balanced.

Real food, made from scratch, leaves you refreshed—not heavy, slug-gish, or uncomfortable.

Vanilla Ice Cream:
A CLEAN TREAT DONE RIGHT

When we want ice cream, we stay loyal to Straus Organic Vanilla.

Their ingredient list is short and refreshing: just organic milk, cream, cane sugar, egg yolks, vanilla extract, and real ground vanilla bean.

Nothing artificial, nothing hidden—just real food.

That's why it stands out to us. Other commercial brands leave a fake aftertaste or a heavy feeling.

But Straus reminds us how satisfying real ingredients can be.

Eating real food restores your natural satiety signals. You no longer crave excess because your body feels nourished at a deep, cellular level.

Homemade Pies:
LEMON TART AND PECAN PIE

Two homemade pies always have a place in our freezer: lemon tart and pecan pie.

- ▸ The lemon tart is simple: eggs, lemon, butter, and sugar—clean, sharp, satisfying.
- ▸ The pecan pie is made the old-fashioned way with brown sugar and butter—no corn syrup, no oils, no gummy gel textures.

These pies don't just taste better—they preserve your digestion, sup-port hormone balance, and protect energy levels.

Our Philosophy:
REAL INGREDIENTS, REAL RESULTS

When making any dessert, I always:
- ‣ Choose recipes with butter, coconut oil, or real dairy—never seed oils.
- ‣ Reduce the sugar when possible without compromising taste.
- ‣ Gravitate toward eggs, whole milk, butter, real vanilla, and organic flours.

Once you start eating foods in their authentic, unprocessed form, you lose the taste for chemical-laden foods altogether. Even nostalgia can't undo it—when I occasionally try a processed treat, I often can't even finish one bite. Your body knows when it's being nourished—and when it's being poisoned.

Homemade desserts support digestion, protect against inflammation, and leave you feeling satisfied without the crash or regret.

The real secret to lasting vitality and youthfulness isn't deprivation—it's in choosing real joy, real flavor, and real nourishment every day.

HEALTHY DESSERTS SUPPORT VITALITY
- ‣ Real fats lower cortisol and improve sleep
- ‣ Lower sugar reduces aging glycation in cells
- ‣ Pure ingredients support skin clarity and digestion
- ‣ Homemade treats nourish natural satiety, not food addiction

Real ingredients. Real indulgence. Real nourishment.

DINNERS FOR DOGS:
FEEDING HEALTH, VITALITY, AND LONGEVITY

Simple homemade strategies for a lifetime of wellness

THE FOUNDATION:
CHICKEN, RICE, AND REAL VEGETABLES

Chicken and rice have been the foundation of our dogs' dinners for their entire lives. Our dogs are now sixteen years old, thriving with health and vitality, and I credit much of that to their real food diet. While they occasionally enjoy table scraps of other meats, their daily dog bowls always include:

- Freshly baked chicken or turkey
- Cooked white rice
- A rotation of fresh, dog-safe vegetables: cucumbers, sugar snap peas, green beans (lightly steamed and frozen in portions), cabbage, summer squash, and butternut squash.

For variety, I alternate their kibble—between a simple chicken formula and a lower-fat fish version. They also receive a thoughtfully selected combination of herbal and mineral supplements to support their digestion, joints, skin, and heart.

WHAT GOES INTO A DOG DINNER BOWL
Here's a glimpse into one of their typical dinner bowls:

- Chicken and/or turkey, chopped into small bites
- White rice (a few teaspoons or tablespoons depending on size)
- Vegetables (small pinches of chopped cabbage, squash, and parsley/cilantro)
- Diatomaceous earth (¼ teaspoon+)
- MSM powder (⅛ to ¼ teaspoon, depending on size)

- ‣ Ground pumpkin seeds (1 teaspoon daily for fiber and minerals)
- ‣ Optional: Homemade chicken broth (1–2 tablespoons)

Everything is prepped fresh or pre-cooked in batches and frozen in easy-to-serve portions—making dinnertime quick, efficient, and joyful for both dogs and humans.

DOG DINNER

- Chicken - prep cooked and cut into pieces
- 1-3 tablespoons of white rice
- Vegetable assortment - squash, cucumber
- Pinch of chopped cabbage
- 1 teaspoon of pumpkin seeds
- chopped parsley and cilantro
- Celtic sea salt - a couple shakes
- MSM 1/8-1/4 teaspoon
- Diatomaceous earth 1/4+ spoon
- Burdrock root - smidge

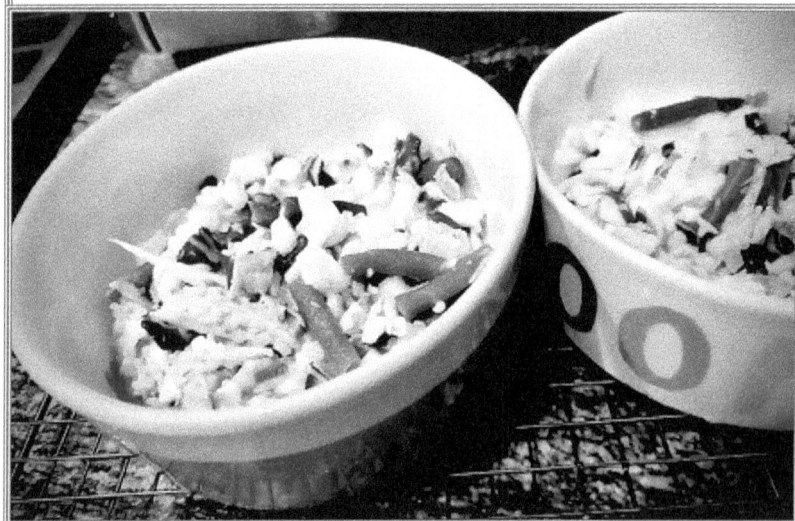

SUPPLEMENT STRATEGIES FOR LONG-TERM VITALITY

We supplement our dogs with many of the same life-enhancing minerals and herbs that we use ourselves.

These additions focus on detoxification, anti-inflammation, circulatory support, and cellular health:

- Diatomaceous Earth: A rich source of silica, essential for connective tissues, bones, and detoxifying heavy metals.
- MSM (A natural sulfur compound that supports joint health, detoxification, and cellular repair).
- Burdock Root: A gentle, nutrient-rich herb known for its blood-purifying properties.
- Hawthorn Berry: A traditional heart tonic that strengthens cardiovascular function safely over time.

When introducing any new supplement, start with the tiniest amount possible—a "smidge" or "drop" spoon is perfect for precision. My dogs are smaller (seventeen and thirty-two pounds), so serving sizes are adjusted accordingly.

(As always, consult your veterinarian before adding new foods or supplements to your dog's diet.)

VISIBLE SIGNS OF HEALTH

Since adding diatomaceous earth and burdock root into their diets, we've seen notable changes:

- Their eye discharge, once persistent, has almost entirely cleared up.
- Their energy, coat condition, and digestion remain vibrant even in their senior years.

It's another reminder that simple, consistent choices—made with care and real ingredients—build true longevity.

BUILDING A STRONGER, HEALTHIER DOG

Simple habits, lasting vitality

▸ Real foods protect digestion, joints, and skin
▸ Herbal support boosts heart, liver, and immune health
▸ Mineral supplementation promotes detoxification and cellular repair
▸ Homemade meals minimize exposure to preservatives, fillers, and harmful additives
▸ Daily consistency creates strength, longevity, and vibrant energy over the years

THE HEART BEHIND EVERY MEAL

Cooking from scratch isn't just about taste—it's about reclaiming control over what goes into our bodies.

Every meal we prepare at home is a decision:

▸ To choose clean, real ingredients
▸ To avoid hidden toxins and preservatives
▸ To build strength, youthfulness, and vitality from the inside out

Yes, it takes more effort. Yes, sometimes it feels like a hundred little steps. But each one of those steps leads somewhere powerful—to better digestion, clearer skin, stronger energy, sharper focus, and a sounder mind.

Choosing real foods, real fats, and natural preparation methods isn't complicated—it's simply built on care, consistency, and the wisdom of real experience. These habits reflect years of refining, learning, and witnessing what happens when you let real food nourish you naturally.

Healthy living doesn't have to be bland, restrictive, or joyless. It can be rich, flavorful, satisfying—and freeing. Every choice you make in your kitchen is a step toward the life and vitality you were designed to live.

After building a foundation of real, nourishing meals, it's just as important to clear out the foods that work against you. Not everything marketed as "healthy" truly serves your vitality or supports anti-aging.

In today's wellness culture, some of the most popular products are cleverly disguised imposters—full of hidden toxins, heavy metals, or anti-nutrients that slowly chip away at health, energy, and sound mind.

The next step in reclaiming your youthfulness, clarity, and strength is knowing what not to eat. Let's take a closer look at the common culprits—and why saying "no" to them is one of the smartest strategies you can make.

Every meal is a decision.
Choose real food.
Build real health.
Eat for the life you want.

The "No" List:
FOODS TO AVOID

Clearing out hidden dangers to protect vitality,
youthfulness, and a sound mind

We've talked a lot about what to add to your plate. Now let's talk about what not to. In today's wellness culture, marketing often outweighs actual nutrition. A product can wear the label "healthy" and still work against your body.

That's why this **"No" List matters**—it's not about fear or perfection. It's about discernment. It's about clearing out the imposters so that real nourishment can take its rightful place.

HIDDEN DANGERS IN "HEALTH FOODS"
Not everything labeled 'clean' is working for you

Many so-called health foods are nothing more than cleverly packaged products that burden the body, confuse the gut, and derail long-term vitality. Anti-aging begins with removing what dulls your glow, slows your mind, or stresses your system.

ENERGY DRINKS:
A CAN OF TROUBLE

Artificial energy comes at a real cost

Let's be honest—if you're reading a health book, you probably already know: energy drinks are toxic traps.

They promise energy but deliver chaos: synthetic caffeine, sugar substitutes, lab-made chemicals, and all of it in aluminum cans. If you're tired, the answer isn't a chemical jolt—it's deeper rest, better nutrition, and blood sugar balance.

Skip the can. Reach for something that actually supports your energy:
- Lugol's iodine or sea kelp for thyroid support
- Organic black coffee for a natural lift
- A blood sugar-stabilizing meal to prevent crashes

Personally, I've never touched an energy drink. They're insidious and hazardous—nothing natural, nothing nourishing.

PROTEIN POWDERS:
PROCESSED AND PROBLEMATIC

Why real food always wins

Protein powders are everywhere—but that doesn't make them healthy.

Yes, they're convenient. But most powders are full of:

- Artificial sweeteners and flavorings
- Thickeners and gums
- Trace toxins and heavy metals
- Isolates your body doesn't fully recognize

The result? Gas, bloating, inflammation, and long-term burden.

Muscles may grow—but true strength includes digestion, clarity, and radiance.

Instead, choose:

- Boiled eggs
- Roasted chicken or turkey
- Leftover clean meat from dinner

These give you bioavailable protein—real nourishment that digests cleanly and supports long-term health.

NUT "MILKS":
A MISLEADING TREND

What you're really drinking—and why it matters

Almond, soy, and oat milks have had their moment. But the truth? They're not milk. They're processed residue.

I used to drink soy milk in my twenties, thinking it was healthy. But once I learned how anti-nutrients affect hormones and digestion,

I stopped. Nut milks are often made from the soaking liquid—the very part meant to be discarded when preparing nuts traditionally.

Now it's bottled, branded, and sold as health food. It's not.

Stick with real milk, ideally organic and whole.

Don't let trends replace real food.

"HEALTH" BARS:
CANDY IN DISGUISE

Convenience at the cost of digestion and vitality

Most bars are just candy with a health halo—loaded with:
- Soy or whey protein isolates
- Refined sugars or sugar alcohols
- Chalky binders, synthetic vitamins, and poor-quality fats

Your body doesn't digest them—it stores the burden and works to detox later. That leads to sluggishness, inflammation, and premature aging.

Better options?
- Hard-boiled eggs
- Roasted pumpkin seeds or macadamia nuts
- Yogurt with homemade preserves
- A small homemade pecan sandie

Clean fuel. Honest food. Lasting energy.

REAL FOOD, REAL RESULTS

Your body recognizes real food—and thrives because of it

The closer food is to its original form, the more your body knows how to absorb it, use it, and benefit from it. Radiance, clarity, energy—they don't come from a can, packet, or processed bar. They come from what grows, what lives, what's whole.

So when you're faced with a quick fix, remember:

Every meal is a choice with impact. Make it count.

CLEARING THE PATH FOR TRUE HEALTH

Every choice either fuels vitality or drains it. This isn't about being perfect—it's about being wise, consistent, and grounded in what works. By clearing out the foods that work against your goals, you open the door to deeper healing, resilience, and long-term strength.

Now that we've cleaned the slate, we'll go deeper into what to build next: targeted, natural supplementation to support real regeneration and cellular health.

Let's keep going—one real strategy at a time.

PART 2

STRATEGIC SUPPORT: SUPPLEMENTS, HERBS & DETOX

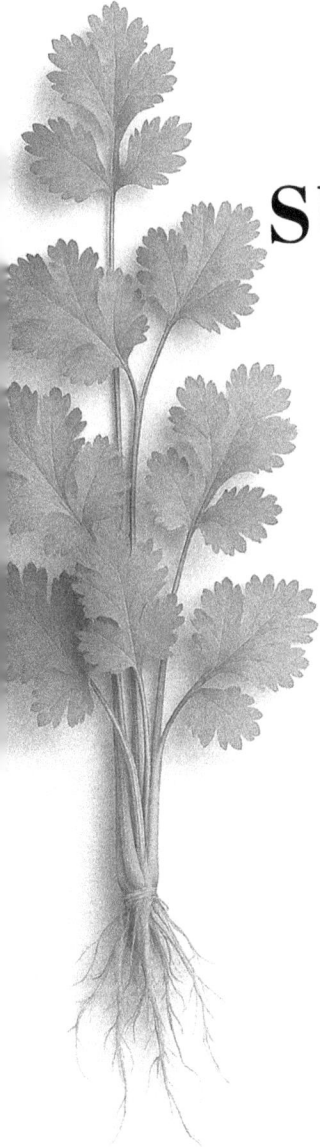

CHAPTER 5

SUPPLEMENTS

Nature's Medicine Cabinet:
ENHANCING HEALTH FROM THE INSIDE OUT

Simple tools. Real results. Healing that starts within.

Supplements have been an essential part of my health journey for many years. I've experimented with it all—capsules, teas, powders—always searching for the most natural, effective ways to build vitality, prevent imbalance, and support long-term resilience.

This chapter isn't a prescription—it's a real-life reflection. These are the remedies I've tested, lived with, and still use to this day. Some worked instantly. Others needed time. And a few, I let go of along the way. But the ones that remain have helped sharpen my mind, restore youthful energy, and support the kind of vibrant, stable health that lasts.

One of my most trusted reference points throughout the years has been the timeless book Back to Eden by Jethro Kloss. It opened my eyes to what our ancestors already knew: Nature is the original pharmacy.

It's not about complexity—it's about clarity. When used wisely, natural remedies are simple, potent, and deeply effective.

What follows is a walk through my personal cabinet—not theory, but tools I live by. These supplements support energy, detoxification, digestion, and skin strength. They're part of how I maintain vitality, year after year—for myself and for my dogs. Let's start with the plants that cleanse: the herbs that keep the body clear, the skin glowing, and the systems moving with ease.

Detox Herbs:
NATURE'S CLEANSING ALLIES

Herbal tools to clear, restore, and renew

Herbs are some of nature's most powerful allies when it comes to detoxification. Whether used daily or seasonally, they work gently but effectively to support the blood, liver, lymphatic system, and skin—the body's natural pathways for cleansing and renewal.

These three standouts have supported my clarity, energy, and glow for years:

RED CLOVER
- Supports blood purification and lymphatic flow
- Helps clear inflammatory skin issues
- Traditionally used to restore radiance and improve skin tone

YELLOW DOCK
- Stimulates bile flow and liver detox
- Enhances digestion and elimination
- Often used to resolve skin issues rooted in internal toxicity

BURDOCK ROOT
- Deeply purifies the blood and lymph
- Known for reducing parasites and biofilm buildup
- Strengthens skin texture—making it less prone to cuts, cracks, and fragility
- Used worldwide as both food and medicine

MY PERSONAL DETOX ROUTINE

In my twenties and thirties, I did seasonal full-body cleanses using those herbs: three capsules of each herb, three times a day, until the bottles were finished. It was a powerful reset. Every time, I felt lighter, clearer, and more stable—physically and mentally.

Today, I focus mostly on burdock root for daily maintenance. It's one of the few herbs that produced visible, lasting results in my skin. I used to get frequent cuts on my fingers—small but annoying. Since using burdock consistently, my skin feels tougher, more elastic, and less fragile overall.

Our dogs take it too. They're sixteen years old now and still vibrant. My groomer often mentions how remarkable it is that they don't have that typical "old dog" cloudy eye. I believe burdock plays a role in keeping their bodies clear and youthful.

GENTLE, ONGOING DETOX IS ANTI-AGING

You don't need to wait for a health crisis to cleanse.

Keeping herbs like red clover, yellow dock, and burdock root in your routine helps your body stay light, radiant, and resilient—from the inside out. They're not quick fixes. They're long-term allies. And when used wisely, they help clear the path for energy, mental clarity, and glowing skin at any age.

CILANTRO:
THE FRESH GREEN POWERHOUSE

Daily greens that detox, digest, and deliver visible results

Cilantro is one of my favorite daily herbs—and not just for the flavor. It's antimicrobial, digestive, and deeply detoxifying, especially when it comes to heavy metals like mercury and aluminum.

That's three foundational strategies for anti-aging—wrapped into one beautiful, fragrant bunch.

KEEPING IT FRESH & FUNCTIONAL

To make sure it lasts, I store cilantro upright in a glass jar with a little water at the bottom, loosely covered with a plastic bag. It stays crisp and vibrant for a full week—ready to use every morning.

I used to rely heavily on leafy greens, especially salads. But over time, I noticed that many lettuces didn't digest well. Cilantro, on the other hand, feels like it works with your body. It stimulates digestion and helps your stomach process food with ease.

Now, when I make a salad, I often skip the lettuce altogether and use crisp veggies and a homemade vinegar and oil-based dressing instead. It's a shift that feels better—and digests better.

HOW WE USE CILANTRO DAILY

Every morning, I chop a few tablespoons of cilantro and sprinkle it over our eggs. The taste is clean, bright, and refreshing. Once you get used to it, you won't want eggs without it. It's amazing to me how underused herbs are at breakfast. I wasn't raised with fresh herbs, but once I started experimenting, they became part of our everyday meals—and the benefits were immediate. Better digestion, better flavor, better energy.

Even our dogs get fresh cilantro sprinkled over their food. It's not just a garnish—it's part of our anti-aging kitchen.

CORIANDER:
THE HEALING SEED OF CILANTRO

Coriander, the dried seed of the cilantro plant, is a regular in our spice lineup. Like its leafy counterpart, it's antimicrobial, digestive, and detox-ifying—especially when it comes to heavy metals and inflammation.

It also brings something more subtle to the table: a warm, grounding aroma and a skin-smoothing effect I've noticed firsthand. When I use coriander consistently—my hands feel noticeably softer and smoother. It's a small detail, but one I can see and feel. That's what makes it worth it.

TANGIBLE RESULTS OVER THEORIES

Anyone can read about what an herb might do.

But when you feel the difference in your digestion...

When you see the difference in your skin...

That's when it becomes part of your life.

Cilantro and coriander have earned their place on my plate—not because they're trendy, but because they work. Every small choice adds up.

And in the world of anti-aging, herbs like these are your quiet, everyday allies.

Real greens. Real digestion. Real glow.

PARSLEY:
A FRESH HERB FOR BREATH AND BEYOND

Small sprigs. Big impact.

Parsley may be one of the most overlooked herbs in modern diets—but in our home, it's a staple. We've eaten it daily for nearly twenty years, and its benefits go far beyond fresh breath.

Yes, it's an excellent natural breath freshener—and yes, our dogs eat it too. We chop it into their meals right alongside cilantro. Their breath is clean, their faces smell fresh, and even the groomer notices. It's like the Febreze commercial, but real life.

But parsley isn't just for breath. It's a quiet powerhouse.

WHY PARSLEY BELONGS IN YOUR ANTI-AGING PLAN
This simple green herb is packed with nutrients that support:
- Kidney health and natural detox pathways
- Heart and brain function
- Blood sugar balance
- Immune strength and mitochondrial protection

- Even potential neuron regeneration—supporting memory and cognitive clarity

That's a whole lot of power in something most people use as plate garnish.

SIMPLE, CONSISTENT, AND HIGHLY EFFECTIVE

We keep parsley fresh just like cilantro—stored in a jar of water in the fridge, loosely covered with a plastic bag. It stays vibrant and ready to chop.

A few sprigs over eggs, a handful in broth, or a spoonful added to any meal—it's a small habit with long-term payoff.

Parsley doesn't demand attention.

But it delivers results you can feel—from the inside out.

Real herb. Real detox. Real resilience.

DIATOMACEOUS EARTH: THE UNSUNG MINERAL THAT DELIVERS

Clean dirt, clear gut, real glow

If I had to pick one underrated supplement that quietly changes everything, it would be diatomaceous earth.

This fine, mineral-rich powder is made from the fossilized shells of microscopic algae—and it's loaded with silica, one of the most essential yet overlooked minerals for anti-aging.

Silica supports:
- Stronger skin, hair, and nails
- Healthy joints and connective tissue
- A resilient gut lining
- Detoxification without stress or strain

We've been using food-grade diatomaceous earth daily for nearly five years, and it's now one of the most grounding, effective tools in our health routine.

HOW WE TAKE IT

In the middle of the day on an empty stomach, I mix 1 tablespoon into 4–6 ounces of water and drink it down. (Using a wooden or plastic spoon)

It's simple. Clean. No frills.

But the effects are powerful:

▸ Helps restore healthy bladder function
▸ Supports digestion and soothes my stomach
▸ Keeps unwanted gut bugs in check
▸ And gives me a light, balanced feeling all day

I've tested this supplement by taking breaks—and every time I do, I notice the difference within days. My stomach feels off, my system slows down, and I don't feel as clear or strong.

Now, it's a non-negotiable. I don't skip it.

PROOF YOU CAN SEE

Even our dogs take it—about ¼ teaspoon mixed into their meals.

One of the first things we noticed? No more runny eye discharge. Their faces became brighter, clearer, and more youthful-looking.

It's not hype—it's visible proof that this "dirt" works from the inside out.

SIMPLE, SILENT, AND SERIOUSLY EFFECTIVE

Diatomaceous earth won't win any beauty contests—but it will help you feel better than almost anything else.

It's one of the simplest ways to detox gently, support your gut, and feed your body the silica it craves for anti-aging strength.

Real minerals. Real results.
Real clean from the inside out.

MSM:
THE DETOX MINERAL
THAT CHANGED EVERYTHING

The simple supplement that gave me my life back

Of all the supplements I've tried, MSM is the one that changed everything. It's an organic sulfur compound—clean, affordable, and incredibly effective.

I was struggling with neuritis and cystitis for over three years. My body felt off—fragile, reactive, and drained. I hit a point where something had to give. That's when I found MSM—and everything shifted. It was like my system recalibrated. The inflammation calmed. My nerves steadied. My self came back.

THE POWER BEHIND THE SIMPLICITY
One of MSM's greatest strengths? It helps detox aluminum, a toxin most people are unknowingly carrying. Aluminum hides in our food, water, deodorants—even the air we breathe. MSM binds to it and helps move it out, gently and consistently.

For me, that detox process made a real difference. My mind felt clearer. My body felt lighter. And my symptoms began to fade.

MY MSM ROUTINE
We now take 8,000 mg daily:
- 4,000 mg powdered in cranberry juice (morning)
- 4,000 mg in capsules (evening)

It's one of the few supplements I refuse to skip.

A QUIET GIANT
MSM doesn't come with hype. But it delivers. It supports:
- Detox
- Joint strength

- Skin repair
- Immune balance

I'm not a doctor—just someone who got her life back. MSM helped rebuild me from the inside out.

Real sulfur. Real strength. Real results.

Parasite Cleanse: REGAINING CONTROL OVER DIGESTION

Simple herbs, major gut reset

We started doing parasite cleanses after noticing just how many lingering digestive issues could be linked to hidden gut bugs. Even with a clean diet, something still felt off—and it wasn't until we addressed parasites directly that everything began to shift.

My husband takes nearly all the same supplements I do, so naturally, this became a shared protocol. And the results were undeniable.

THE HIDDEN CULPRIT BEHIND DAILY DISCOMFORT

In my experience, many stomach issues are bug-related—even if you're eating well. Parasites, fungi, and pathogenic bacteria can quietly take root, creating subtle, chronic imbalances that interfere with digestion, energy, and clarity.

The classic parasite cleanse uses three herbs:
- Black walnut
- Wormwood
- Cloves

It's a simple, three-week protocol—no complicated diets, no harsh restrictions. Just capsules, taken consistently.

I first started it during my cystitis recovery, and it couldn't have been easier to integrate. But what happened afterward was the real surprise.

BEFORE THE CLEANSE: SUBTLE SIGNS WE MISSED

Before we ever knew what was going on, we noticed something strange: We couldn't eat sweets unless we also ate nuts. If we had a chocolate chip cookie without cashews, our stomachs would be wrecked. Even dairy started to cause bloating and discomfort.

We didn't recognize it at the time, but these were classic signs of microbial imbalance. The gut was off—and our bodies were trying to manage it any way they could.

THE CLEANSE AND THE SHIFT THAT FOLLOWED

Once we introduced parasite cleansing—alongside MSM and diatomaceous earth—everything changed.

Stomach upset went from daily to rare.

If something does flare up now, we know exactly how to address it—quickly and naturally.

At first, we did the full cleanse every four months for a year. Now, we maintain as needed—maybe once or twice a year. These herbs have become staples in our cabinet, and we don't go without them.

THE PARASITE-FIGHTING TRIO

WORMWOOD: STRESS RELIEF + MICROBIAL BALANCE

Wormwood is deeply calming—physically and mentally. It's anti-fungal, antimicrobial, and helps rebalance gut bacteria. When digestion feels off—grumbling, bloating, discomfort—a few wormwood capsules usually bring quick relief.

BLACK WALNUT: NATURE'S HEAVY HITTER

One of the strongest anti-parasitic herbs available. It's also antiviral, anti-fungal, and rich in omega-3s. I take it a couple times a week for maintenance—and bonus: I've noticed my hair looks healthier and more vibrant while using it regularly.

CLOVES: SWEET RELIEF AND DAILY DEFENSE
Cloves are antimicrobial, antioxidant-rich, and great for digestion. If I eat something sweet or feel too full after a meal, I take cloves to settle things down. They've become a daily insurance policy for gut comfort and immune support.

STAPLE HERBS FOR A CLEANER, STRONGER GUT
This trio—black walnut, wormwood, and cloves—is simple, natural, and deeply effective. In a world full of processed food and hidden pathogens, these ancient tools help us stay clean, resilient, and strong from the inside out.

Real herbs. Real cleansing. Real gut control.

CAYENNE PEPPER:
POWER FOR DIGESTION, CIRCULATION, AND IMMUNE STRENGTH

A natural stimulant that lights up your system from the inside out

Cayenne pepper is one of the most potent healing tools I've used—and one of the simplest.

Its benefits reach across the body: stimulating digestion, boosting circulation, supporting immune strength, and even improving oral health. For me, it started as a focused effort to heal from cystitis and ended up becoming a daily habit that radically improved my overall vitality.

HOW I DISCOVERED CAYENNE'S POWER

During my cystitis healing journey, I was determined to clear out anything that didn't belong—parasites, fungus, candida, or bacterial overgrowth. I wanted natural solutions that worked.

I came across a YouTube video where a man shared how nothing had worked until cayenne. He said cayenne was the only thing that reached deep enough to make a real difference. He took large doses and described how his energy, clarity, and gut stability returned—almost like a reset. He made one thing clear: you may not be able to completely eliminate parasites, but you can weaken them, control them, and reclaim your health.

That inspired me to try cayenne. I started with capsules at each meal—and I haven't looked back since.

DAILY USE: FIVE YEARS AND COUNTING

I've taken cayenne capsules with nearly every meal for over five years, and my digestion has never felt better. It helps my body break down food efficiently, prevents bloating, and gives me a steady, internal warmth that feels like a circulation boost from the inside out.

Cayenne doesn't just help the gut—it stimulates blood flow, which in turn supports oxygen delivery, nutrient absorption, and even detoxi-fication. It's a wake-up call to the system.

CAYENNE, STRAIGHT UP

A few years into my cayenne use, I discovered the work of Dr. Barbara O'Neill. Her approach to cayenne was even more direct: drinking it in water.

Following her example, I began adding 1/4 teaspoon of cayenne to a glass of water, especially on days when I wanted an extra boost. You can literally feel the heat traveling through your bloodstream—sometimes all the way to your ears. It's not uncomfortable—it's invigorating. You can feel something shifting, flowing, waking up. It's a natural vitality enhancer that costs pennies a day.

UNEXPECTED BONUS: DENTAL AND ORAL HEALTH

One of the most surprising benefits I've noticed since drinking cayenne water is the improvement in oral hygiene. I've had less plaque and tartar buildup—and at times, it has disappeared entirely when I'm consistent.

Why? Because drinking cayenne in water hits your mouth and throat directly, neutralizing harmful bacteria before they make it to your gut. It's an easy, effective way to support oral health naturally—something many people overlook when focusing only on digestion.

BEST PRACTICES & TIPS

- Capsules: Always take with food and plenty of water. If you don't, you may feel intense stomach heat or irritation. (If that happens, just drink more water—it passes quickly.)
- Cayenne Water: Surprisingly, drinking it on an empty stomach has never caused me discomfort. When your taste buds sense the spice, your body seems to activate digestion correctly—proof of how intelligently designed our systems truly are.

NATURAL POWER YOU CAN FEEL

Cayenne is not a trendy supplement—it's an ancient powerhouse with modern relevance. Whether taken in capsule form or mixed into water, it delivers a noticeable boost in energy, circulation, immunity, and digestive strength.

It's simple. It's effective. And it's one of the few tools that gives you instant feedback: you feel it working.

Real spice. Real heat.
Real results that keep your system strong,
youthful, and flowing freely.

GINGER:
ANCIENT SPICE FOR DIGESTION, IMMUNITY, AND INFLAMMATION

A daily root for deep, lasting vitality

Ginger is one of the most powerful medicinal foods in nature—and one of the easiest to enjoy.

This timeless root is a digestive stimulant, antimicrobial powerhouse, and natural anti-inflammatory. It supports immunity, soothes the gut, and helps the body fight off bacterial, viral, and fungal infections—all while adding a warm, grounding flavor to your day.

Studies even show ginger may protect the liver, reduce oxidative stress, and support cardiovascular health. But in our home, the benefits go far beyond the research—we feel them firsthand.

HOW WE USE IT DAILY

Each evening, we brew fresh ginger tea—a simple routine that's become one of our favorite rituals.

Here's what we do:

▸ Peel and cube fresh ginger
▸ Add 1–2 teaspoons of the chopped root into a small thermos
▸ Fill with boiling water and steep for 1–2 hours
▸ Pour into small glasses and sip slowly after dinner

The result is a rich, spicy, soothing infusion that calms digestion, boosts circulation, and helps the body wind down. If we want a deeper hint of ginger's heat and healing, simply chew a small piece of the infused ginger. It's sharp—but effective. Just a bite can help ease bloating, stimulate enzyme activity, and support immunity.

THE POWER OF SIMPLICITY

Ginger doesn't need hype. It's stood the test of time—used across generations and continents as a trusted remedy for everything from nausea to inflammation. It's simple, accessible, and remarkably effective.

Whether sipped, steeped, or chewed, ginger is a daily ally in supporting your digestive strength, immune function, and anti-aging energy.

Real root. Real fire. Real everyday medicine.

Seeds:
SMALL BUT MIGHTY

God-given nourishment for energy, clarity, and lasting strength

Seeds are one of God's simplest, yet most powerful creations.

Each one is a tiny life source—packed with nutrients, designed to grow and sustain life. They're not manufactured in a lab or processed into synthetic forms. They were built into the earth by design—to restore the body, preserve youth, and renew the mind.

When we include seeds in our daily routine, we're not just snacking—we're activating restoration.

These humble powerhouses remind us that God already provided what we need to thrive: real foods that protect health, support clear thinking, and help us age with grace.

APRICOT SEEDS: A TREND THAT FADED

Years ago, apricot seeds were popular in alternative circles, especially for their rumored anti-cancer benefits. We tried them ourselves, but their extreme bitterness made them difficult to enjoy—and impossible to sustain. While they may still have a place in some protocols, we chose to move on and focus on seeds that offer both benefit and usability in real life.

CARDAMOM: A BREATH OF FRESH AIR

This ancient seed is well-loved in Chinese and Ayurvedic medicine for its digestive and antimicrobial properties. Cardamom supports the heart, liver, urinary tract, and even brain function. We occasionally chew 5–6 whole seeds, which freshen breath while quietly supporting internal health. I've even shared a few granules with our dogs for an herbal breath boost.

ANISE SEED: THE SWEET HELPER

Anise is another timeless herbal seed—great for digestion, immunity, and inflammation. Its sweet, licorice-like flavor makes it easy to enjoy. I sometimes use it in baked goods or take a pinch straight for sore throats or stomach relief.

CORIANDER SEED: A SOOTHING CLASSIC

Coriander, the dried seed of the cilantro plant, has long been used to support digestion, blood sugar balance, clearer skin, and even eyesight. I sprinkle it on our eggs every morning. And I've noticed: when I use it consistently, my hands feel softer and less dry. That's the kind of subtle, lasting impact that shows a seed is truly working.

FENNEL SEED: GENTLE AND REFRESHING

Fennel is both soothing and stimulating. These little seeds are anti-inflammatory, antimicrobial, and excellent for digestion and respiratory health. Chewing a few seeds throughout the day freshens the breath naturally while gently enhancing clarity and calm.

SESAME SEEDS: ANCIENT SUPPORT FOR HORMONES AND HEART HEALTH

With over 3,500 years of use behind them, sesame seeds are rich in calcium, magnesium, zinc, and healthy fats. They've been shown to support hormonal balance, blood sugar regulation, stress reduction, and even respiratory function.

I keep it simple—sprinkle them over eggs, soups, or roasted vegetables. Their mild, nutty flavor goes with nearly everything, making them an effortless way to nourish the body, every day.

SMALL SEEDS, LASTING STRENGTH

It's easy to overlook something so small—but inside each seed is a world of nourishment. They help regulate digestion, cleanse the body, support brain health, and contribute to vibrant energy and glowing skin.

These are not trends—they're timeless tools, placed here by God to fuel our systems gently and effectively. When we lean into what He provided in its purest form, we often find the strength, clarity, and youthfulness that no synthetic formula can match.

The answer to vibrant health often starts small—just like a seed.

Real Seeds. Real Nourishment. Real Strength.

▸ Packed with life-sustaining nutrients
▸ Support digestion, brain clarity, and strong immunity
▸ Natural tools for youthful energy and resilience
▸ Proof that sometimes, the smallest foods have the greatest power

HERBS & HORMONES

Natural support for balance, beauty, and lifelong vitality

Keeping your hormones in balance is a cornerstone of feeling vibrant, youthful, and strong—at every stage of life. Whether it's sleep, skin, energy, or mood, your hormones set the rhythm. And the good news? You don't have to rely on synthetic options to support them. Balanced hormones benefit everybody—and natural strategies can go a long way.

Herbs offer a real, God-given way to restore balance naturally.

They're not quick fixes—but when used consistently, they can shift how you feel from the inside out.

I pay close attention to how I feel before and after introducing any new supplement or food. Subtle sensitivities are often tied to hormonal fluctuations. Your body speaks—listen closely.

As I've navigated hormonal changes (especially those related to estrogen loss), I've explored herbs that gently support the transition. Some work through the nervous system. Others act through digestion, detox, or mineral balance. But all of them share one thing: they offer real results without disrupting the body's natural design.

ROSEMARY: A DAILY HORMONE HELPER
Rosemary became a daily staple after I baked a homemade rosemary bread in a cast iron skillet. The way we both felt after eating it consistently—more balanced, vitalized, and clearer—led me to dig deeper.

Rosemary supports:
- Hormone regulation
- Cognitive clarity
- Digestion and detox
- Hair strength
- Mood and circulation

But what really stood out? My night sweats vanished. Since adding rosemary regularly, I haven't had a single episode. That's how subtle shifts can lead to powerful outcomes.

My quick method? Butter on a tortilla chip, sprinkled with rosemary. Easy. Delicious. Life-improving

BLACK COHOSH: GENTLE RELIEF FOR DEEPER REST
I turned to black cohosh after struggling with disrupted sleep that felt hormone-driven. Castor oil helped, but only temporarily. Black cohosh changed things.

From the very first dose, my sleep deepened—longer, more restful, and more dream-filled. It felt like a switch had flipped.

This herb is known to:

▸ Ease hormonal tension
▸ Reduce inflammation and spasms
▸ Calm the nervous system
▸ Support restful sleep

It became one of my favorite hormone allies—not flashy, just effective.

RED CLOVER: ESTROGEN SUPPORT + GENTLE DETOX

Red clover has long been used as a blood purifier and lymphatic cleanser—but it's just as useful for balancing hormones during transition.

Its benefits include:

▸ Mild estrogenic support
▸ Improved circulation
▸ Bone and cardiovascular strength
▸ Gentle detox and skin clarity

I take it as a tea or in capsule form when I'm on the go. Either way, it's a steady tool in my herbal rotation—especially when I want to feel balanced and nourished.

SESAME SEEDS: ANCIENT HORMONE NUTRITION

These little seeds have stood the test of time—over 3,000 years of use in ancient health traditions. They offer gentle hormonal nourishment for both women and men.

In women, sesame seeds support healthy estrogen levels. In men, they've been linked to fertility and testosterone regulation. For both, they contribute to mineral balance, stress resilience, and heart support.

I sprinkle sesame seeds over my eggs in the morning—an easy, every-day hormone helper.

RESTORING BALANCE THE NATURAL WAY

Hormones touch every part of your life:

Energy. Skin. Sleep. Mood. Weight. Memory. Confidence.

As we age, nurturing them with herbs is one of the kindest things we can do for our bodies. Herbs aren't magic—but they are powerful. They offer gentle, grounded support that works with the body—not against it.

Herbs were built into creation to help the body thrive—meant to nourish, protect, and support its natural rhythms. When used with intention and consistency, they become part of a lifestyle that fuels long-term vitality and lasting glow.

Real herbs. Real harmony. Real anti-aging power.

Fish Oils:
A MIXED REVIEW

Questioning the hype—and trusting real-life experience

Fish oil supplements are everywhere—touted as essential for heart health, brain function, joint support, and inflammation control. The message is loud and clear: "You need your omega-3s."

But over the years, I've learned that what works on paper doesn't always translate into real-life results.

I'm still not sold on fish oils.

RANCID OILS, MALE HEALTH RISKS & THE UNKNOWNS

Fish oil capsules have a reputation for going rancid quickly—even before they reach your shelf. And once they oxidize, they don't nourish the body —they burden it. Some research even links fish oils to potential negative effects on men's hormone and prostate health, which made me pause before ever handing them to my husband.

We've gone most of our lives without taking fish oil—and we've done just fine. I'm not interested in risking long-term damage from unstable fats or hidden additives, especially when the benefit is still debatable.

FRESH FISH ISN'T ALWAYS SAFER

The usual fallback is to just "eat more fish." But that opens another issue: Heavy metals. Mercury. Environmental toxins.

We tried incorporating sardines daily for a short stretch—and while they seemed okay, it was canned mackerel that tipped the scale. Almost immediately, we both felt toxic and foggy. Even our dogs—who had small servings—started acting tired and melancholy, with a haze in their eyes. We cut the fish, and everyone bounced back.

That experience taught me this:

Even "natural" sources can backfire if they're not clean.

ANECDOTES VS. SCIENCE

It's true—some people swear by fish oil. I have a friend whose doctor doubled his dose and saw his cholesterol drop dramatically. That's intriguing.

But I've also seen studies that say the opposite—warning of oxidative stress, hormone disruption, or diminished returns. Everyone seems to have data to back their angle.

MY PERSONAL VERDICT? CAUTION OVER CONVENTION

These days, we eat fish occasionally—maybe a shrimp cocktail here or there. But we've stepped back from the hype. I'm not against fish oils—but I'm not jumping in blindly either.

There's wisdom in observing. Trying something for yourself. Noticing how it feels. Because even the cleanest supplement might not align with your body in the context of everything else: your hormones, your age, your stress, your baseline.

SOMETIMES LESS IS MORE

In a world overloaded with supplements and theories, fish oils remind me that more isn't always better. Your body knows. Watch, listen, and trust your own response.

Fish oils. Mixed results. Proceed wisely.

THE TEA TABLE:
A DAILY PRACTICE FOR DETOX, BALANCE, AND VITALITY

A cup of calm. A habit of healing.

Tea is more than a beverage—it's a daily anti-aging ritual.

Whether steeped in the morning light or sipped in the quiet of evening, herbal tea offers one of the simplest, most powerful anti-aging practices you can adopt. It engages the senses, hydrates the body, delivers real plant medicine—and brings clarity and focus in a world that rarely slows down.

WHY I DRINK TEA EVERY DAY

Unlike capsules or tinctures, tea invites you to slow down and receive. You smell it. You taste it. You feel it warming your core. And with every sip, it delivers therapeutic compounds that help detox the liver, soothe inflammation, regulate hormones, and cleanse the body.

It's restoration in liquid form. Real tea is consistent and designed to nourish—not overstimulate.

CHOOSE QUALITY. CHOOSE SIMPLICITY.

When possible, I stick to single-herb, organic teas—brands like Traditional Medicinals, Buddha Teas, and Choice. The simpler, the better. When you brew just one herb at a time, you get to know its character. Its flavor. Its effect on your body. And over time, you'll sense which herb your system needs most on any given day.

MY FAVORITE ANTI-AGING TEAS

JAPANESE GREEN TEA

This is my antioxidant-rich favorite. Lightly caffeinated, yet calming.
It supports:
- Cardiovascular health
- Blood vessel protection
- Mental clarity and circulation

At restaurants, I'll order green tea with a side glass of ice—a refreshing, refined way to stay aligned with clean living while eating out.

YELLOW DOCK TEA

This is my detox hero. It supports:
- Liver health
- Lymphatic flow
- Parasite and microbial elimination

It's earthy, bold, and you can feel it working. I've even given this in powder form to support my senior dog's liver function. If it's healing for me, it's healing for them.

NETTLE & RED CLOVER TEA

A powerful duo for:
- Hormone balance
- Detoxification
- Mineral nourishment
- Circulation and skin clarity

These teas aren't just for women—men benefit, too. They support natural energy, joint comfort, and overall vitality.

DANDELION TEA (OCCASIONAL)

While it's a classic detoxifier, we learned firsthand that dandelion can cause reactions in some people. My husband developed soreness and tightness in his hands after regular use—so we now reserve it as an occasional cleansing tea.

It's a great reminder: even good things aren't one-size-fits-all. Always listen to your body.

DAILY TEA, DAILY DETOX

Drinking herbal tea is one of the most effective ways to support detoxification, hormone harmony, digestion, and immune function. And you're not just flushing out toxins—you're infusing your body with plant-based strength that supports every organ system.

In a world full of distractions and chemicals, tea offers something different: a slow, sensory reset that works with your body—not against it.

LET IT STEEP. THEN LET IT TRANSFORM YOU.

Tip: Choose high-quality organic single-herb teas whenever possible to fully experience the flavor, purity, and health benefits nature intended.

Real tea. Real medicine. Real anti-aging results.

LOWER CORTISOL,
SLEEP BETTER, AGE STRONGER

Simple, natural strategies to restore rest, rebuild resilience, and keep your glow

Sleep is one of the body's greatest repair mechanisms—and one of the first things to slip as we age. Whether it's falling asleep, staying asleep, or waking too early, sleep disruptions become more common—and more frustrating.

Mainstream advice pushes pills, sleep gummies, or nightly Benadryl. But if you've chosen a natural path, you already know: real sleep doesn't come from synthetic fixes. It comes from restoring your body's rhythm.

At the center of most sleep struggles? Elevated cortisol—the stress hormone. When cortisol is high at night, your body stays wired. Lower it—and sleep follows.

FAT BEFORE BED: A GAME-CHANGER

One of the most effective tools I've ever used for sleep is eating fat before bed. It may sound too simple to work—but it does.

I first heard this from Dr. Elizabeth Bright, who suggested a tablespoon of butter before sleep—and again if you wake in the night. It was a turning point.

Personally, I often use a tablespoon of extra virgin olive oil instead. Both methods work.

They help:

▸ Lower cortisol
▸ Stabilize blood sugar
▸ Signal the body it's time to rest—not stay alert

Bonus? Fats like butter and olive oil don't just help you sleep—they keep your skin youthful.

Real fat nourishes the cells from the inside out—fewer wrinkles, less dryness, and deeper overnight repair.

Sleep deeper.
Wake restored.
Age better.

St. John's Wort:
CALM IN A CAPSULE

When my nervous system feels too "on," I reach for St. John's Wort. It's a natural cortisol-reducer that helps the mind and body downshift—fast.

We take it in capsule form, and the results were noticeable from day one. That wired tension from high cortisol? Gone. Replaced with a steady calm that actually lasts.

Known for centuries as a mood-stabilizing herb, St. John's Wort helps:

- Ease nervous tension
- Quiet mental overactivity
- Promote restorative sleep
- Reduce that edgy, irritable feeling that can creep in as hormones shift

My husband noticed the difference too—calmer evenings, smoother transitions into sleep, and waking up feeling more grounded.

SLEEP THAT BUILDS YOU BACK UP

When you lower cortisol, you don't just sleep—you restore. You wake with clarity. You handle stress better. Your skin glows again. This is how real anti-aging works—through the night, while your body rebuilds.

Small, consistent strategies like these create lasting changes in sleep quality, mood stability, and overall vitality.

Nature's tools are simple—but their impact is profound.

Real rest.
Real repair.
Real results.

VITAMINS:
FOUNDATIONAL SUPPORT FOR LASTING VITALITY

What you absorb shapes how you age

Supplements aren't side notes in my health routine—they're strategic tools I use every day to maintain energy, clarity, and long-term resilience. But not all vitamins are created equal—and not all of them work in your favor.

QUALITY OVER QUANTITY

When it comes to vitamins, I only use clean, hypoallergenic, high-quality brands. My go-to is Thorne—trusted for purity, precision, and real results. I stick to capsules over tablets because they absorb better and contain fewer fillers.

Too many popular supplements boast high potency but deliver a fraction of what they claim. Independent tests have shown it—and most people never know. But it matters. Immensely. If you're serious about your health, quality isn't a luxury—it's a requirement.

WHY I ALSO PRIORITIZE HERBS

Herbs aren't just an "extra" in my routine—they're a core piece of the foundation. They deliver living nutrition, not just isolated vitamins. Herbs support detoxification, regulate hormones, feed the nervous system, and bring balance where the body needs it most.

One of my favorite local stores, Herbally Grounded, says it best:

"Herbs are your real vitamins." I still use Thorne's precision formulations, but I always weave in herbs—because together, they create a complete support system for lasting vitality.

MY CORE SUPPLEMENT ROTATION

I rotate my supplements to keep the body adaptive and responsive. Here's a look at what stays in steady rotation:

- Thorne Basic Nutrients 2/Day
- Men's/Women's Multivitamins
- Thorne Vitamin B Complex
- Thorne Vitamin C
- Thorne Vitamin E
- Thorne Vitamin D
- Thorne Zinc + Copper
- Boron + Vitamin K
- Curcumin
- Cayenne Pepper (with every meal)
- Black Walnut + Burdock Root
- Fish Oil (New Chapter—when used)

Supplements are active agents—never neutral.
Every pill you take either builds strength or adds burden.
Choose with clarity. Choose with purpose.

SUPPLEMENTS ARE SERIOUS TOOLS

- Pick brands that prioritize purity and potency
- Choose capsules for better absorption
- Rotate your supplement routine to stay balanced
- Use herbs like living vitamins—they're nature's originals
- Remember: Real health starts with real ingredients

MAGNESIUM STEARATE: AN ADDITIVE TO AVOID

Watch what's hiding in your "health" supplements.

Just because a label says "vitamin" doesn't mean it's clean.

So many store-bought supplements are packed with hidden additives that reduce effectiveness—or worse, interfere with your body's ability to absorb the good stuff.

Magnesium stearate is one of the most common culprits. It's a flow agent used during manufacturing—but it can actually reduce absorption and block nutrient delivery.

I've made it a rule:

If I see magnesium stearate or maltodextrin, I put it back on the shelf.

I want pure, single-ingredient supplements.

For example, I buy a pure MSM powder with zero fillers.,

REAL-WORLD EXAMPLE

A friend of mine started taking MSM to help with brain fog and was loving the results. Then he bought a different brand—and the results disappeared. Why?

We flipped the bottle and saw the difference: magnesium stearate.

It makes a difference.

CLEAN LABELS, CLEARER RESULTS

Every time you take a supplement, you're either supporting your body—or asking it to work harder.

A clean label usually means better absorption, fewer reactions, and more visible, lasting results.

Always read the fine print. It's where your health lives.

- ‣ Supplement Smarts: Watch for Fillers
- ‣ Magnesium stearate: flow agent that may block absorption
- ‣ Maltodextrin: often GMO and blood sugar disruptive
- ‣ Choose clean, single-ingredient options whenever possible

EVERY CHOICE BUILDS THE FOUNDATION

Supplements aren't magic pills.

They're tools—powerful ones—when chosen with discernment.

Every capsule, every herb, every mineral is either:

- ‣ Building your resilience
- ‣ Or silently working against you

This chapter isn't about chasing trends or blind faith in marketing.

It's about building youthfulness with intention.

It's about saying no to fillers, shortcuts, and fakes.

It's about choosing what truly fuels your body to thrive.

The supplements you take today are shaping the version of you that shows up tomorrow.

You're building your future one capsule at a time.

Make every choice count.

Pick clean. Stay sharp.
Build resilience from the inside out.

CHAPTER 6

THE FAST

APPLE JUICE CLEANSE:
THE RESET THAT WORKS

Real cleanse. Real clarity. Real energy.

THE CLEANSE THAT DELIVERS

Fasting is everywhere right now—especially intermittent fasting. And while skipping breakfast might have its benefits, this isn't that. This is a real, full-body reset: five full days of targeted cleansing to clear the gut, calm inflammation, and wake up your senses. My husband and I first did this cleanse nearly 25 years ago. It wasn't trendy. It wasn't pretty.

But the transformation? Unforgettable.

We felt lighter, brighter, and unbelievably sharp. Even touch felt heightened—like our bodies had just rebooted.

THE APPLE JUICE / COLON CLEANSE PROTOCOL

I stumbled across this cleanse online, long before detoxing was a trend. What caught my eye?

Pictures. Rubbery, rope-like waste coming out of people's intestines. Not normal bowel movements—deep intestinal buildup.

Skeptical but curious, I ordered a simple powdered mix of psyllium husk and bentonite clay—two natural binders known to pull toxins and debris from the digestive tract.

The protocol is simple but powerful:

- Drink only apple juice (5–6 servings a day)
- Add psyllium + bentonite powder
- Hydrate with water between each round

We started with bottled organic juice from Trader Joe's—and yes, it worked. But later, we leveled up.

THE FRESH JUICE ADVANTAGE

Once we switched to fresh-pressed apple juice, everything intensified.

The living enzymes, the natural acids, the flavor—it took the cleanse into high gear.

We'd grab 4–6 containers a day (32 oz each) from a local juice bar or press it ourselves. The difference is real.

We prep using empty 16 oz plastic water bottles—perfect for shaking, not stirring.

Psyllium thickens fast, so every round gets a fresh bottle.

And between each juice dose? One full bottle of clean water—to keep things moving.

Bonus tip: add a dash of cayenne to boost circulation and heat things up.

WHAT TO EXPECT EACH DAY

Day 1: Manageable. You're adjusting to the cleanse. Stay distracted and sip consistently.

Day 2: Rough. Cravings hit hard. You might feel foggy, tired, moody, or even irritable. This is the detox wall—rest and push through.

Day 3: Energy starts to return. You'll notice a lightness and mental clarity creeping in.

Day 4: You're in the zone. The brain fog lifts, hunger fades, and you feel clean and focused.

Day 5: Full adaptation. You're barely thinking about food. You feel alert, light, and deeply restored.

And yes—the rubbery buildup came out.
It was real. And honestly? It was empowering.
You realize how much has been sitting inside—and what your body feels like without it.

SENSORY RESET. MENTAL LIFT. CELLULAR CLARITY.
This cleanse goes beyond digestion.
It clears the fog. Sharpens your hearing. Heightens every sense.
Colors feel brighter. Sounds are crisper. Your skin glows. Your hugs feel electric.
It's not subtle—it's a full-body reactivation.

TIPS & TOOLS
‣ Powder: Psyllium husk & Bentonite clay
‣ Juice: Fresh-pressed is best. Organic bottled if needed.
‣ Cayenne: 1/8 tsp for blood flow
‣ Frequency: Every 3 hours. Water in between.
‣ Tools: 16 oz bottles for mixing—easy shake, no clumps

RESULTS THAT LAST
After years of consistent cleansing, I had a colonoscopy.
The doctor looked at me and said,
"You have the colon of a poster child for perfect health."

I wasn't surprised. This cleanse has been our annual reset—and it's delivered every time.

We do it once a year, without fail.

Because when something makes your body feel clean, alive, and plugged back in—you don't forget it.

You build your health around it.

IF YOU TRY IT...

Be prepared. You'll need commitment.

But if you give it five days—fully—you might just feel like a new person.

Not just lighter. Not just clearer.

Rejuvenated. Connected. Complete.

Real cleanse. Real clarity. Real energy.

This isn't a trend.

It's a reset that rewires how you feel in your body—and how you age from here on out.

CLEANSING CHECKLIST

- **Fresh apple juice (5–6 14 oz./day—space at the top for shaking):** The main fuel—rich in enzymes and malic acid to support liver function.
- **Psyllium husk and clay blend:** Natural binders that grab and eliminate old waste (1 teaspoon psyllium husk, 1/4 teaspoon powdered bentonite clay).
- **16 oz plastic water bottles:** Essential for quick mixing—psyllium thickens fast.
- **Filtered water (daily):** Aim for a full 16 oz between each juice round to keep things moving.
- **Cayenne pepper (optional):** A dash (⅛ tsp) in some rounds can boost circulation and digestive fire.

- **A light schedule:** Plan light activity—especially on Days 2 and 3. Stay home if possible.
- **Commitment:** Five days. No shortcuts. The transformation is worth it.

Real cleanse. Real reset. Real transformation.

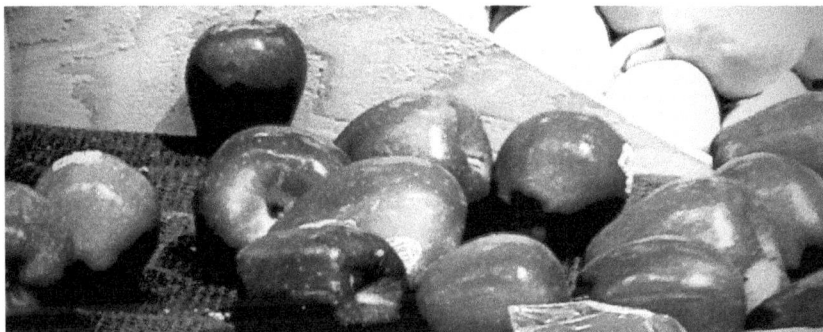

Reset your system.
Recharge your body.
Reclaim your health.

PART 3

MOVEMENT & DAILY MAINTENANCE

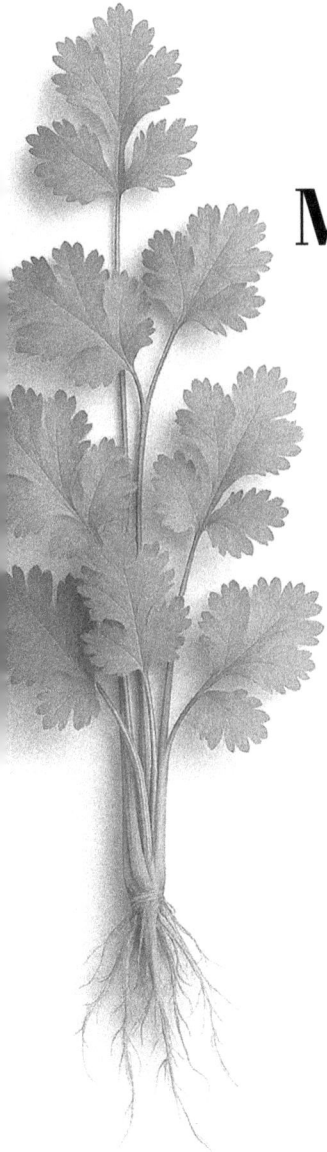

CHAPTER 7

MOTION

MOVE IT OR LOSE IT

Motion is non-negotiable if you want to stay young. I've believed this since my early teens—and I live it now, in my mid-50s. If your blood isn't moving, your health is stalling. Movement builds energy, sharpens your mind, clears your skin, strengthens your heart, and keeps your body running like it should. It's the foundation of vitality.

It all started with a simple bike ride around the lake. The fresh air, the sweat, the mental reset—it felt amazing. That feeling stuck. I didn't wait for motivation; I created momentum. Now, movement isn't a chore—it's a built-in strategy for anti-aging, hormone balance, and brain clarity. And the key is consistency. I work out every week. No exceptions.

I've used a treadmill for decades. I sprint now instead of long runs, and I've added backward walking with the machine off—it works muscles you don't hit going forward and builds full-body strength. I also rebound—bouncing on a mini trampoline—to stimulate my lymphatic system and reduce inflammation. No equipment? No problem. Do jumping jacks. Jog in place. Move.

Even on vacation, I stay active. At a campground, I'll jog the trails. In an airport on a long layover, I walk the terminals. In Kentucky, I've jogged past white fences and horse farms just to start my day with a boost. It's not a sacrifice—it's a pick-me-up.

Movement oxygenates the blood and awakens the body. It elevates your mood and sharpens your mind. When I was young, I saw older people losing their strength and agility, and I thought, 'If I keep doing it, maybe I'll always be able to do it.' That logic has kept me moving—and it's paid off.

The truth is simple: Move it, or lose it.

No Excuses Movement: Simple Ways to Stay Active Anytime

- *Rebounder* – 5–10 minutes a day stimulates your lymph system
- *Walk the airport* – Make layovers productive
- *Backwards treadmill steps* – Low impact, high benefit
- *Jumping jacks* – 50 reps, no equipment needed
- *Morning jog* – Even 10 minutes clears the mind
- *Sprints* – Add 3–5 to your treadmill for a youthful boost

Consistency beats perfection. Just move.

Move it. Feel it. Keep it.

Your strength, your youth, your energy—
they all depend on motion.

STRETCHING:
DAILY FLEXIBILITY FOR LIFELONG AGILITY

Stretching isn't just a warm-up or cooldown—it's a powerful anti-aging tool. If you want to stay youthful, flexible, and pain-free, stretching is essential. The same principle applies here as with movement: if you keep doing it, you'll keep being able to do it. But if you stop, stiffness and restrictions start to settle in. Flexibility is a form of freedom—and one that must be maintained with consistency.

One of the most important ways to maintain a youthful, upright posture is by keeping your muscles elongated. A full range of motion isn't just for athletes. It's for anyone who wants to bend down, reach high, twist, turn, and move through life with ease. Stretching supports circulation, realigns the body after a day of repetitive postures, and helps keep you tall, open, and balanced.

The more consistently you stretch, the more likely you are to preserve your full range of motion. And when you move with ease, you feel youthful. Why limit your motion when you can expand it? When you stretch regularly, your spine stays tall, your shoulders remain open, and your chest stays lifted.

MORNING & NIGHT STRETCHING

Start your day with light, energizing stretches to awaken circulation and set the tone for movement. Evening stretches are restorative—perfect for releasing built-up tension, relaxing the nervous system, and improving sleep quality. I find that stretching before bed is essential. Our bodies go through so many static positions during the day; stretching resets everything to keep alignment, ease, and comfort in place.

STRETCHING SUPPORTS DETOX

Stretching doesn't just help you stay limber—it also supports detoxification. Moving and elongating the muscles stimulates lymphatic flow, which helps flush toxins from the body. That's why even light movement—like a simple stretch session or a few deep intentional movements can leave you feeling clearer, calmer, and more refreshed.

THE STRETCHES I USE DAILY

- ▸ Toe Touch: A simple forward bend stretch can help loosen tight hamstrings, lengthen the spine, and improve circulation in just a few breaths. This is the baseline. Can you touch your toes? If not, start today and build up. It's an easy way to stay limber.
- ▸ Gentle Backbend Stretch: Lie flat, then lift your chest while keeping your hips grounded. It's a great way to open the chest, strengthen the spine, and increase circulation. I used to do this

stretch daily without thinking. Then I stopped—until I realized how tight my midsection had become. Now it's back in rotation.

▸ Lying Twist Stretch: One of my go-to moves for releasing tension. Just lie on your back, pull one knee across the body, and let your spine gently unwind. It's simple, effective, and feels incredible after a long day.

▸ Neck and Shoulder Mobility Work: I like to start with a few gentle shoulder-loosening rotations and neck release movements—just enough to shake off any stiffness and restore flow. These help release built-up tension from stress or screen time.

▸ Joint Mobility Circles: rolling the wrists and ankles—can help wake up your circulation and keep smaller joints flexible as you age. Don't forget the small joints—keeping them mobile prevents stiffness over time.

Stretching isn't just maintenance—it's momentum. It keeps your joints nourished, your posture proud, and your entire body in youthful alignment. The more often you engage, the longer your vitality lasts.

Don't wait until you're stiff to start stretching.
Daily mobility is long-term vitality.

Neck Stretches:
STRENGTHEN, SCULPT, AND STAY YOUTHFUL

While many people focus on core, legs, or even posture for anti-aging benefits, neck stretches are one of the most underrated tools for staying youthful—both in function and appearance. The neck is one of the first areas to show signs of aging, and keeping it strong and mobile can help maintain firmness, blood flow, and skin tone.

A simple daily stretch of moving your head forward and backward helps increase circulation to the neck muscles. This enhanced blood flow not only helps with mobility but supports skin health and muscle tone, keeping sagging at bay.

For deeper impact, I've tried more advanced movements like laying on your back with your head over the edge of the bed. Let your head slowly hang back, then bring it forward again. You can also do this standing—hold a hand weight to stabilize your body as you tilt your head gently backward and return to center.

Another staple is neck rotations. Rotate your head in full, slow circles—three times in one direction, then three in the other. These help loosen tight muscles, prevent stiffness, and promote youthful skin by stimulating blood flow in a key area.

Your neck matters. Don't ignore it in your routine. A few intentional minutes each day can firm your skin, boost circulation, and keep your posture strong and youthful.

Neck stretches improve circulation, reduce stiffness, and protect against sagging.

COMPOUND MOVES: ANTI-AGING POWER IN EVERY REP

If you want to stay young, strong, and flexible—compound exercises are non-negotiable. These are the movements that work multiple muscle groups at once, keep your joints healthy, and challenge your coordination. They don't just build muscle—they build longevity.

SQUATS: YOUR FOUNDATIONAL YOUTH MARKER

The deep squat is one of the most telling indicators of aging—and one of the easiest to reclaim. Before chairs, this was the default rest position. Now, most people can't even get into it without discomfort. But if you can squat—and stay there—you're preserving mobility most people lose with age.

I started squatting while hanging out with the dogs. Now it's habit. Anytime I have a minute, I drop into a squat. My feet are flat. My hips are open. This one move keeps your knees, ankles, and spine agile. Work up to it. Your body will thank you.

Add in other squats and lunges to activate more muscles. Try narrow-stance squats, wide-stance, and walking lunges. These compound movements engage multiple muscle groups at once, increasing blood flow and coordination—making them some of the most efficient exercises you can do.

PUSH-UPS: THE ALL-IN-ONE STRENGTH TEST

Push-ups engage your arms, chest, core, and back in a single, powerful motion. Even one a day builds strength. It's the easiest, most portable way to stay strong—and it costs nothing but commitment. No equipment. No excuses.

If you're short on time and can only pick one movement for the day, this is the one. Push-ups build strength, stamina, and discipline.

CORE CONTROL: THE CENTER OF POWER

I skip sit-ups. Leg lifts and planks do more for your abs with less risk to your back. These movements stabilize your spine, tone your waistline, and keep your posture tall and lean. You'll look better, move better, and age better with a strong core.

These aren't fancy exercises—they're primal movements your body was designed to do. They're how you preserve strength, power, and functionality well into your later years. You don't need a gym. You need motion, discipline, and a few minutes a day.

THERAPY ACCESSORIES FOR CIRCULATION AND MUSCLE RELIEF

KEEP THE BLOOD MOVING, KEEP THE BODY YOUNG

One of the simplest ways to stay youthful, vibrant, and mentally sharp is to keep your blood flowing. Good circulation is at the core of good health. It nourishes your cells, detoxifies your tissues, and even sharpens your mind. God designed the body with intricate systems that thrive on movement—and when we support those systems, everything works better. Using basic therapy tools like rollers and massage balls helps stimulate blood flow, release tension, and encourage the kind of internal movement that keeps us looking and feeling young.

ROLLING FOR RELIEF

For promoting circulation and working out stiff or sore muscles, there are countless tools available—and many of them you can use right at home. My personal favorites are back rollers in a variety of sizes. Foam rollers, textured rollers, and even homemade solutions can be incredibly effective.

I simply roll my back out on the floor, using different tools depending on the area I want to target. Legs can be rolled too, and it's a simple way to bring blood flow into tired or tight muscles. I've collected an assortment of rollers and balls over the years to address different pressure points and tension areas.

BALL-BASED MASSAGE TOOLS

My first massage ball was a basic tennis ball. Chiropractors often recommend it because it's accessible and effective. Most suggest standing against a wall while rolling to control pressure, but I prefer the floor—it gives deeper pressure. However, the added body weight can be too intense if you're not careful. Be mindful and listen to your body so you don't overdo it.

Over the years, I've experimented with all kinds of massage balls:

- Tennis ball: great starter for general use
- Golf ball: excellent for pinpoint pressure work
- Volleyball: offers a gentler stretch, especially across the shoulder area

I lie on my back and gently roll over each ball to stimulate specific areas. There are countless pressure points you can reach this way, and it's an empowering way to take charge of your own muscle care.

THE SPIKED BALL

One of the simplest and most effective tools is the spiked massage ball—about the size of a tennis ball but covered in firm, rounded spikes. It's an excellent stimulator for the feet and the top of the head. Use it in any direction to activate circulation and bring fresh blood flow into stagnant areas. It's quick, effective, and feels incredible when used mindfully.

DEEP ROLLING SUPPORT

If you're looking for something beyond foam rollers, the Chirp Wheel set is a fantastic option. These come in a set of four sizes, each designed to maneuver between the shoulder blades and along the spine. The smallest wheel works well for targeted tension, while the largest provides a full back stretch from shoulders to hips. They're built with just the right firmness to offer deep pressure without discomfort.

A NOTE OF CAUTION

While these tools can be highly effective, remember that more pressure isn't always better. The floor allows for a deeper massage, but it also increases the risk of overdoing it. If you're new to self-massage or physical therapy tools, it's wise to consult your doctor or a physical therapist before starting. Be gentle, pay attention to how your body responds, and approach each session with care.

WHERE BLOOD FLOWS, LIFE FOLLOWS

When blood flows freely, everything in the body improves—skin glows, joints move with ease, and the mind stays clear. These simple therapy tools may seem small, but they help wake up areas of the body that need attention. They encourage circulation in places where it's slowed down or stuck, bringing life back into tired muscles and stagnant tissues. And with that improved circulation comes better oxygenation, better brain function, and a better sense of well-being. God gave us what we need to stay strong and sharp—sometimes we just have to get things moving.

A MOVING BODY IS A LIVING BODY

Movement isn't just exercise—it's preservation. From walking and stretching to rebounding, squatting, or using simple therapy tools, every motion is an investment in youthfulness, strength, and mental clarity. A body in motion keeps its circulation strong, its joints flexible, its muscles toned, and its mind sharp.

Whether you're sprinting on a treadmill, stretching before bed, rolling out tight muscles, or just walking through an airport terminal instead of sitting—every step, bend, and breath is a reminder: you are choosing vitality. You are choosing a younger, stronger, more resilient version of yourself.

Keep moving. Keep choosing life. Because a moving body isn't just alive—it's thriving.

Keep moving. Stay strong. Age with purpose.

CHAPTER 8

TOPICAL HEALTH AND BEAUTY

From Head to Toe: SKINCARE YOU CAN TRUST

TOPICAL HEALTH THAT REFLECTS INTERNAL VITALITY

Your skin is your largest organ—and it deserves the same care and quality you give your diet. If you wouldn't eat it, why let it soak into your body? That's my standard now.

After years of experimenting with traditional skincare, I realized most products left my skin puffier, more irritated, and ultimately less youthful. Fragrances, fillers, emulsifiers—most creams on the shelf are chemical cocktails. They might feel smooth, but what are they doing beneath the surface? I don't want temporary plumpness that masks deeper damage. I want real results: vibrance, clarity, and strength that lasts.

That's why I switched to edible-grade ingredients—simple, pure, and effective. Products I could literally eat if I had to.

*"If it's not clean enough to eat,
it's not clean enough for your skin."*

FACE SKINCARE:
REAL FATS, REAL RESULTS

SIMPLE INGREDIENTS FOR TIMELESS SKIN

Your face is one of the first places aging shows up—and one of the best places to show off the glow of good health. That's why I stopped chasing expensive creams with ingredient lists I couldn't pronounce and started feeding my skin the same way I nourish my body: with clean, whole fats.

It all began with shea butter—pure, rich, and uncomplicated. I used it on my face, hands, and dry spots for years. But then I discovered tallow. Fatworks makes a beautiful lamb tallow that glides on silkier than shea butter and sinks into the skin like it belongs there. For around $14 a jar, it lasts forever and completely replaced my need for conventional skin creams.

Here's the secret: healthy fat heals.

Tallow is naturally antimicrobial, making it a protective, nourishing base for the skin. It doesn't need preservatives or synthetic fillers. My mild rosacea improved. Redness faded. My skin became calmer, more balanced—just from using real, edible-grade fat.

Then I met castor oil.

I thought it would be too thick—but it's been a game changer. It clears blemishes, softens tone, and adds a glow that no commercial serum has ever given me. And no, it doesn't clog pores. Quite the opposite—it soothes, heals, and restores.

MY NIGHTLY FACE PROTOCOL:
- A fingertip of lamb tallow
- A few drops of castor oil
- Gentle massage to boost circulation and skin tone

That's it. Clean, potent, and powerful.

Even my husband uses this combo. He's in his sixties, and I've noticed a real difference in his skin—smoother, brighter, more youthful. Proof that this isn't just for women. It's for anyone who wants skin that reflects health from the inside out.

No fragrances. No emulsifiers. No empty promises.

Just fats your skin recognizes, and results you can see.

Pure ingredients. Real skin. Natural beauty, no filter.
"Ditch the chemicals. Feed your skin what it craves—
pure fats, no fillers, all glow."

FACIAL CLEANSERS & MASKS

Purity Over Products: Cleaning Your Face Without Compromise

When it comes to facial care, I don't rely on overpriced cleansers with 25 ingredients I can't pronounce. I've used the Trader Joe's Oatmeal Bar Soap for years. It's simple, unscented, and made with a short, clean ingredient list. You don't need harsh chemicals to keep your face clear and glowing—just consistency and purity.

I don't wear foundation or trend-based cover-ups. I'm not interested in makeup that clogs pores and masks the natural tone of the skin. A real anti-aging strategy means keeping your skin healthy enough that you don't need to cover it up in the first place. A clean face is a youthful face—one that reflects the health underneath.

A CLASSIC THAT STILL WORKS

For detoxifying and minimizing pores, I use the Queen Helene Mint Julep Masque. This clay-based mask has been around since 1930, and there's a reason it's lasted this long—it works. It draws out impurities, clears the skin, and leaves it smooth and refreshed. I used it as a teen, and I'm still using it decades later.

There's no overpowering scent, no trendy marketing fluff—just a solid product that helps reset your skin. After I use it, I always follow up with a few drops of castor oil and a dab of lamb tallow to replenish moisture and restore balance. Together, they soften the skin, improve texture, and maintain that youthful glow.

Real Skin. Real Simplicity. Real Results.

PURE PROTECTION: CLEAN HANDS WITHOUT COMPROMISE

Real Ingredients. Radiant Skin. Everyday Defense.

In a world hyper-focused on staying germ-free, hand sanitizer has become a staple—but most commercial formulas are far from health-supportive. Laced with synthetic alcohols, artificial scents, and chemical binders, these "protective" gels often deliver more harm than help. They dry out the skin, disrupt the microbiome, and introduce toxic compounds into the bloodstream through daily use.

The same concern applies to typical liquid hand soaps. One glance at the label reveals a lineup of unpronounceable ingredients that serve the manufacturer more than the consumer. These soaps are often made with harsh detergents, drying alcohols, and chemical fragrances—all of which strip your skin's natural oils, damage your barrier function, and speed up the visible signs of aging.

For someone like me, whose skin is ultra-sensitive, the consequences were immediate and painful: cracked, bleeding hands just from using mainstream soap. That was my wake-up call. I made it a non-negotiable to carry my own soap and moisturizer everywhere I go—and I've never looked back.

WHAT I USE INSTEAD

Oatmeal & Honey Bar Soap – Trader Joe's
This simple bar soap has minimal ingredients and never irritates. It cleanses gently, keeps my skin smooth, and doesn't leave behind a film or scent. A staple in my routine.

Dr. Bronner's Pure Castile Soap – Unscented
This is my go-to liquid option. Whether I'm at home or on the road, it's easy to bring along and use. I prefer the unscented version, but the scented ones made with essential oils are still light years ahead of what's on most shelves.

NATURAL MOISTURIZERS:
LAMB TALLOW & OLIVE OIL

For hydration and protection, I skip the synthetics and use what nature provides. I carried shea butter for years, but recently switched to lamb tallow, which feels smoother and delivers deeper moisture. It's antimicrobial, anti-aging, and works perfectly in a travel-sized container.

For an extra layer of protection, I use straight olive oil, the same cold-pressed, organic oil I cook with. It absorbs beautifully, nourishes the skin, and acts as a natural antibacterial agent thanks to its fat content.

ANTI-AGING STARTS AT YOUR FINGERTIPS
Your hands show your age faster than almost any other part of your body. Why speed up that process by coating them with chemical residues all day? Natural, fat-based soaps and moisturizers support skin resilience and hydration—two essentials for keeping hands looking and feeling youthful. The more we simplify, the better our results. Fewer ingredients. Fewer toxins. Fewer cracks, irritations, and signs of wear. These clean choices aren't just gentle—they're powerful.

LIP GLOSS:
REAL MOISTURE WITHOUT THE TOXINS

Why I Ditched the Chemicals for Natural Radiance

There are endless lip products on the market—but are any of them actually good for your lips? Honestly, not many. Lipsticks, in particular, are often a cocktail of synthetic dyes, preservatives, and endocrine disruptors. Most smell artificial, taste worse, and leave your lips drier than before. Those trendy high-shine gloss tubes? They've done little more than mess with my hormones and leave a sticky chemical film behind.

I've found that most lip color, no matter how clean the marketing, still dries out the lips. And yet, like many women, I kept applying it anyway—sacrificing comfort for color.

MY SIMPLER LIP ROUTINE
Eventually, I pared things down. I use basic lip pencils—many of which, thankfully, don't have that offensive odor or chemical taste. They let me define and enhance my lips without the overload. But the dryness was still an issue.

That's where natural fats came in.

I began using coconut oil, which helped with chapped lips, especially in dry weather. But I got even better results when I switched to lamb tallow and castor oil. These deeply moisturizing, single-ingredient products offered nourishment that commercial balms never could. I keep a few small ramekins on my counter with tallow and castor oil—easy to access and apply throughout the day when I'm not wearing color.

No stabilizers. No scents. Just pure, absorbable moisture your body can recognize and respond to.

THE BEST OF BOTH WORLDS
The only downside? I could only use these pure fats when I wasn't wearing lip color—until I found something that worked beautifully alongside my usual routine: a tallow-based lip gloss.

It comes in a classic gloss tube, glides on effortlessly, and blends beautifully with my lip pencil—without breaking it down or drying it out. It's unscented, unflavored, and deeply hydrating. Whether you're wearing makeup or going bare, this gloss delivers real nourishment with zero toxins. It's hands down the best lip gloss I've ever used—and yes, it's great for men too.

EYE MAKEUP REMOVER

Clean Eyes. Clean Ingredients. Clean Conscience.

When it comes to removing eye makeup, the market is flooded with chemical-laden solutions that are anything but skin-friendly. Most commercial removers are filled with synthetic ingredients that don't belong anywhere near your eyes—or your bloodstream. Even the products labeled "gentle" often contain petroleum derivatives and artificial preservatives.

My standard? If I wouldn't eat it, I'm not putting it on my face.

That's why my favorite remover is simple: organic coconut oil. The same Nutiva coconut oil I cook with becomes part of my evening skincare ritual. It melts makeup effortlessly, nourishes the delicate eye area, and supports healthy, blemish-free skin—all without the toxic aftermath.

MY CLEAN MAKEUP REMOVAL ROUTINE:
▸ Plug in my stainless steel mug warmer
▸ Let a small steel cup of coconut oil melt while I wind down
▸ Dip a cotton ball into the melted oil, squeeze off excess
▸ Gently wipe away the day

Coconut oil is naturally antibacterial and antimicrobial. It helps prevent clogged pores and breakouts—unlike many synthetic removers that leave behind chemical residue. Best of all, it feels soothing, not oily. Just clean, calm skin.

WHY I LEFT OTHER OILS BEHIND

Like many others, I started with baby oil. But that's just mineral oil—refined petroleum. Total toxin. Then I tried jojoba, which worked well but wasn't food-grade. I moved on to grape-seed oil, which was better (and affordable), but eventually switched back to coconut oil due to concerns about excess omega-6 intake. I even gave olive oil a try—but the sting near the eyes made that a quick no.

At the end of the day, coconut oil just makes sense. It's a saturated fat your body recognizes. It moisturizes while it cleanses. It supports your natural beauty instead of hiding it behind chemicals.

THE BIGGER PICTURE: NATURAL BEAUTY IS ANTI-AGING

True beauty isn't about fads or fillers. It's about supporting your skin and body with what it actually needs—real nutrients, clean fats, and non-toxic choices. Every time you remove your makeup with something healing instead of harmful, you're casting a vote for vitality over damage.

Say no to chemical cleansers. Say yes to glowing skin—naturally.

Real fats. Real purity. Real beauty.

SKIN TAGS & MOLES:
WHEN BEAUTY CALLS FOR BACKUP

Let's talk about the beauty blemishes no one wants to admit they notice: skin tags, moles, and those odd little growths that seem to pop up with age. I'm not one to let nature have the final say—especially when simple, natural methods can help reclaim a smoother, more youthful appearance.

Years ago, I came across a video of someone using apple cider vinegar to shrink and remove small growths. Intrigued, I tried it. The results?

Real and repeatable. But before you dive in, a quick reminder: always check with a doctor or dermatologist first to rule out anything serious. I have a dermatologist who's frozen off a few skin tags here and there, but sometimes they dismiss them as "nothing to worry about." Maybe so medically—but I still don't want them on my face, neck, or chest.

Here's the protocol I followed:

- Pour a small amount of apple cider vinegar into a ramekin
- Dip a cotton swab and apply it directly to the spot
- Hold for 10–20 minutes, re-dipping frequently to keep the area saturated
- You may feel a slight sting—that's a good sign
- Repeat daily for several days until it scabs, then allow it to fall off naturally

I've done this on spots along my hairline, the side of my nose, even my chest and back. If the spot is thicker or flesh-toned rather than pigmented, I sometimes gently poke it with a clean needle before applying vinegar to help it penetrate. Yes, it gets red. No, it's not pretty at first. But in a couple of weeks? Clear, smooth skin.

Important notes:

- Don't do this the day before a big event—give yourself some healing time. It could take a week or two
- Skip foundation or cover-up while it's healing—just let the process work
- Be extra careful with the face. Try a test spot first
- As always: I'm not a doctor, and this is not medical advice—just what worked for me

Sometimes you don't need a prescription. You just need persistence, a plan, and a little pantry power.

NETI POT:
THE FORGOTTEN HERO OF SINUS HEALTH

There's nothing youthful about chronic congestion, puffy eyes, or sinus infections that linger for weeks. That's why I've kept one simple tool in my arsenal for decades: the Neti pot. It's an old-school solution that still holds up—and unlike a lot of "modern fixes," it's gentle, inexpensive, and highly effective.

I first started with a water pick-style device that had a sinus attachment. It blasted saline water through the sinuses using strong pressure. And while it worked for a while, it always came with a risk: too much force. You could accidentally push an infection deeper instead of clearing it. That's when I switched to the Neti pot—and never looked back.

WHY I PREFER THE NETI POT

The Neti pot works with gravity, not pressure. It allows warm saltwater to flow gently through one nostril and out the other, clearing congestion, flushing out allergens, and helping prevent sinus infections before they take hold. It's proactive hygiene for your head—especially helpful during allergy season, dry winters, or whenever your immune system needs extra support.

MY SIMPLE ROUTINE:
- ▸ Start with a clear glass for each nostril
- ▸ Add enough sea salt to lightly coat the bottom
- ▸ Pour in filtered water, then top with boiling water to warm it
- ▸ Stir well, then test the temperature—it should be warm, never hot
- ▸ Pour into your Neti pot and flush each nostril fully

You'll be amazed how much lighter and clearer you feel afterward. I used to do this every day—especially during cold season—until I started making homemade nasal sprayers. But even now, I keep the Neti pot close. It's my go-to whenever things feel stuffy or off balance.

WHY IT'S ANTI-AGING

Clear breathing, reduced inflammation, and fewer infections all mean less strain on the body. And less strain = more vibrance. It's not just about sinus health—it's about keeping every system flowing, including your lymphatic and immune systems. When your body isn't congested, your skin glows, your eyes brighten, and your head feels clearer.

Sometimes the most powerful remedies are the ones you've had all along.

NOSE STABILIZER:
SMALL DETAIL, BIG IMPACT

Anti-Aging Starts at the Center of Your Face

One subtle sign of aging that's often overlooked is the nose. Yes, the nose. As we age, it's common for cartilage to continue growing, and for some, that results in a broader or more pronounced nose. For me, it started with irritation and unexpected changes around the nasal area—especially after prolonged mask-wearing. I noticed puffiness, and even tiny growths forming. My thought? I'm not letting my nose get bigger without a fight.

My first instinct was to trace it back to bacteria. The nose is a high-traffic area for microbes, and internal inflammation can reflect on the outside. So I turned to one of my favorite universal solutions: raw apple cider vinegar. Of course, I couldn't put it on the outside of my nose—too harsh and too red. But the inside? That was my strategy.

MY ROUTINE

Each evening, I dip a Q-tip into raw apple cider vinegar and gently swirl it inside both nostrils. Just a quick motion around the interior edges. The result? Reduced puffiness, a cleaner nasal passage, and no more unexplained soreness. Bonus: The Neti pot is occasional instead of daily.

And for those who struggle with that seasonal sore nose—the one that feels swollen and lingers for weeks? Apply the vinegar with a cotton swab right to the irritated area, even multiple times a day. Most people see a dramatic improvement within 24–48 hours.

WHY IT WORKS

- Apple cider vinegar is antimicrobial, anti-inflammatory, and balancing
- Regular application helps reduce nasal swelling and surface-level bacterial growth
- It supports sinus health and can reduce the need for nasal rinses
- Keeping your nose in check helps retain facial proportion—a subtle but essential part of anti-aging

Small routines like this one may seem minor, but they accumulate into visible results. Looking youthful isn't just about serums and creams—it's also about keeping inflammation at bay and staying consistent with smart, clean, targeted care.

Small habits. Smart prevention. Youth preserved.

Nasal Sprays:
DAILY DEFENSE FOR CLEAR BREATHING

When it comes to staying vibrant, clear nasal passages are underrated. Chronic congestion, shallow breathing, and recurring sinus pressure all chip away at energy levels, mental clarity, and overall radiance. That's why I've created my own set of daily nasal sprays—simple, natural, and highly effective.

It started one day when I felt a sinus infection creeping in—despite my usual Neti pot routine. I hadn't had one in years, and I wasn't about to let it happen. A coworker shared that she had cured her sinus issues by flushing her nose with apple cider vinegar in a Neti pot. She said it burned, but it worked. I appreciated the tip—but I wanted something more manageable for daily use.

THE SPRAY SOLUTION THAT CHANGED EVERYTHING

That's when I started making my own nasal sprayers.

I bought a couple of empty 2-ounce glass mist bottles. One I filled with warm sea salt water (the same solution I use in the Neti pot). The other? A mix of filtered water and apple cider vinegar—about 1/8 to 1/4 teaspoon per bottle, depending on your tolerance. It sounds mild, but the results are anything but.

That vinegar sprayer is the real deal.

I use both sprays daily. The sea salt sprayer is a great maintenance flush. The vinegar one is more intense—perfect for when things feel stuck, stuffy, or on the verge of infection. If one or two sprays don't do the job, I keep going. I've had stubborn days where I sprayed up to thirty times in five minutes. It stings a little, but it clears the passages beautifully—and breathing returns, clean and free.

MORE NATURAL TOOLS WE USE

My husband occasionally uses a store-bought nasal spray with an iodine blend—clean label, no questionable additives. I keep one on hand too, and it works well. It's a solid option if you're not ready to make your own, but still want to ditch the toxic over-the-counter steroid sprays.

WHY IT'S ANTI-AGING

Breath is life. Clear nasal passages mean better oxygen intake, better sleep, and less inflammation. When you breathe well, everything works better: your brain, your mood, your skin. These natural sprayers aren't just sinus solutions—they're daily detox tools for better vitality.

No pharmaceuticals. No rebound congestion. Just clarity, simplicity, and control.

Breathe Better.
Live Clearer.
Stay Radiant.

Real clearing. Real power. Real prevention.

DITCHING ALUMINUM:
MY SWITCH TO CRYSTAL SALT DEODORANT

I used to think deodorant was just one of those everyday products you didn't question. You bought whatever smelled nice and kept you dry, right? But once I began paying closer attention to ingredient labels—really reading them—I realized I didn't want aluminum salts near my lymph nodes every single day.

The more I cleaned up my health routine, the more I questioned why I was rolling a chemical paste onto my underarms without thinking twice. That's when I found the Crystal salt deodorant stick—a simple, unscented mineral bar made of natural potassium alum.

This wasn't some trendy clean beauty pick. It was solid, pure salt. And surprisingly, it worked. The stick goes on wet, like a water swipe across the skin. It doesn't mask odor with fragrance—it prevents the bacteria that causes odor in the first place. There's no residue, no stickiness, and best of all—no aluminum compounds clogging my pores.

HOW I USE IT
After showering, I dampen the tip of the crystal and glide it gently under each arm. That's it. It dries in seconds, leaves no scent, and keeps me feeling fresh all day. On especially hot days, I'll reapply if needed, but most of the time I don't have to think about it.

It's lasted me years—literally. Unlike traditional sticks that run out every couple months, my first crystal deodorant stick lasted well over a year before I had to replace it.

WHY IT'S AN ANTI-AGING CHOICE

This isn't just about smelling good. Lymphatic flow, hormonal health, and detox support are all tied to what we put near our glands—especially in areas like the underarms. Choosing aluminum-free deodorant is one of the simplest, quietest anti-aging moves you can make. It's not flashy, but it reduces toxin exposure over the long haul. That matters.

By avoiding synthetic fragrances and aluminum, you're minimizing your chemical load, supporting natural perspiration, and letting your body detox the way it was designed to. You're also respecting your skin's barrier instead of confusing it with parabens, triclosan, or talc.

WHAT TO KNOW

- Don't expect artificial dryness. Crystal deodorant doesn't block sweat—it works with your body's rhythm instead of against it.
- Give your body time to adjust. If you're switching from conventional deodorant, your body may purge some odor-causing buildup in the first few days or weeks. Stick with it—it's worth it.
- Stay consistent. Just like any natural remedy, its power lies in steady use, not overuse.

TOENAIL FUNGUS:
THE FIGHT FOR CLEAR NAILS

What Finally Worked After Everything Else Failed

Toenail fungus isn't glamorous—and it's definitely not something people talk about openly. But it's more common than you'd think. When it hit me, I started noticing skin lifting from the nail bed. It wasn't pretty, and I wasn't going to ignore it.

I ditched the toenail polish, rolled up my sleeves, and got serious. I assumed it'd be a quick fix. Wrong. This became one of the longest health experiments I've tackled—and I tried nearly everything.

WHAT DIDN'T WORK

Apple Cider Vinegar
This was my first go-to. I knew it was anti-fungal, and soaking the feet in it made sense. But the amount I'd need regularly would cost a fortune. Dabbing it on helped a little, but not enough to move the needle.

Tea Tree Oil
It had that promising first-day effect. But long term? Nothing changed. And if something doesn't show visible results, I don't stick with it.

Hydrogen Peroxide
I soaked each toe for five minutes. It felt nice at first—clean, fizzy, hopeful. Then the skin started itching and flaking. That experiment ended quickly.

Vitamin C Paste
I even got creative—mixing powdered vitamin C with water into a paste while watching TV. Rinsed it off afterward. Not harmful, just ineffective.

$40 Store-Bought Topical
Easy to apply, and marketed well. But after two months with zero change, I wasn't about to keep buying tiny bottles of wishful thinking.

WHAT ACTUALLY STARTED TO WORK

Baking Soda: Alkaline, Affordable, Effective

This is where things turned. I added a spoonful of baking soda to a small dropper bottle, filled it with water, and applied it to each nail—morning and night. Refreshing, clean, cheap, and anti-fungal. I even made a spray version for quick use. Bonus: it helps raise your alkalinity and feels like a mini reset every time.

THEN CAME THE GAME CHANGER: IODINE

I stumbled on a Dr. Berg video recommending povidone iodine for fungus. I was already familiar with iodine and liked the idea. The solution was thick, stayed on the nail, and I began seeing real results. Eventually, I upgraded to a purer, liquid iodine. No mess. No staining. I used a small dropper bottle and applied it directly—clean and simple.

That's when the breakthrough happened.

My nails started growing back clear. Normal. Healthy.

TOPICAL IODINE FOR DOGS

A Natural Approach to Shrinking Tumors

(Disclaimer: Always consult your veterinarian. This is my personal experience, not medical advice.)

I originally started buying iodine to offset the effects of goitrogens—foods like cabbage and radishes, which we were eating daily. These vegetables can suppress thyroid function when consumed in excess, so my husband and I began using Lugol's iodine to support our thyroid health. Just a few drops each morning became part of our routine—and the dogs joined in too. I simply drop a small amount on a piece of chicken and they eat it with no fuss.

But what really surprised me was what happened when I began using iodine externally—on my dog's skin.

Years ago, one of our previous dogs developed several tumors late in life. Despite feeding him what we thought was a healthy diet, the growths became overwhelming and uncontrollable. That experience stuck with me. So when our current dog began showing signs of developing multiple tumors and raised growths, I knew I had to act fast.

I started with castor oil, which I use regularly on myself. But my dog had a skin reaction to it—so that was out. Then I had a realization: I was already using iodine topically on my own nails… why not try it on her?

SIMPLE ROUTINE, NOTICEABLE RESULTS

I began applying just a few drops of iodine directly onto a different growth every couple of days. It's not a dramatic routine. No bandages, no fancy tools. Just clean hands, a calm dog, and a few drops rubbed gently onto the area.

Yes, it slightly discolors her fur, but it doesn't seem to bother her at all—and the color washes out easily.

What matters most is this: the tumors are shrinking.

She had a mass near her rear that was about the size of a golf ball. Now, it's nearly flat. Another one on her front thigh measured around four inches long and one inch wide. It's noticeably thinner and continues to recede.

She remains calm during every application, and I'm honestly amazed by the progress. This simple, natural step feels like it's making a real difference—not just for her physical health, but for our peace of mind.

Real care. Real sweat. No chemicals.
That's the kind of clean that actually lasts.

BEAUTY IN BALANCE

True beauty doesn't come from a bottle—it radiates from a body in balance.

By simplifying what I put on my skin and choosing ingredients as clean as what I'd put on my plate, I've created a skincare routine that actually supports my health, not sabotages it. Rich fats, edible oils, and minimal products have given me better results than any trending serum ever could.

You don't need twenty products or toxic fillers to age well. You need clarity, consistency, and the courage to go back to the basics.

Less clutter. More glow. That's beauty, the real way.

Feed your skin like you feed your body.
Fewer products. Cleaner ingredients.
That's the real glow-up.

> *"Your skin isn't asking for more products.*
> *It's asking for fewer toxins."*

Glow comes from nourishment, not overload.

CHAPTER 9

HOME SPA

SOAKS AND WRAPS. SWEAT IT OUT.

External Detox Rituals for Internal Renewal

A nti-aging isn't just about what we eat or the supplements we take—it's also about how we treat our body from the outside in. Our skin is a powerful organ of elimination, and if we want to maintain vitality, clarity, and that unmistakable youthful glow, we have to support the body's natural detox pathways at every level.

This section covers the external rituals I personally use to encourage real-life wellness and cellular rejuvenation—from foot soaks and castor oil wraps to my go-to baking soda body spray. These simple, grounding practices help clear the lymphatic system, relax the nervous system, and refresh the skin—while reducing the toxic load that modern life throws at us daily.

These aren't luxury spa treatments or complicated hacks. They're accessible, effective, and rooted in everyday consistency. And over time, they help preserve that ageless look we're all after—clear skin, calm nerves, sharp focus, and a body that stays vibrant.

HOME SPA: SOAKS AND SWEATS
FOR DETOX AND REJUVENATION

Cleansing your body doesn't stop at what goes in—it includes what comes out. Detox isn't just a digestive process; it's a full-body experience. Your skin is your outer shield, your detox gatekeeper, and a daily communicator of your internal health.

Youthfulness is more than skin deep. It's the ability to feel grounded, energized, and pain-free in your own body. That kind of radiance doesn't come from wishful thinking or expensive treatments. It comes from consistent rituals that support your body's built-in systems—practices like sweating, soaking, and skin therapies that encourage release, repair, and regeneration.

Modern life is full of exposures—from processed food and polluted air to blue light and chemical products. If you're not giving your body a consistent outlet to expel what it absorbs, you're not fully detoxing. That's why these home spa strategies matter. They aren't indulgences. They're essentials.

This chapter shares the real-life therapies I depend on to feel lighter, sleep deeper, think clearer, and look younger. Because radiant health isn't reserved for spa days—it's built right at home, one intentional soak or wrap at a time.

"True beauty begins with what you release. Sweat, soak, and let go—because detoxing isn't vanity. It's vitality."

Don't just cleanse—command your glow.
Real radiance starts with release.

Detox Soaks:
THE HEALING POWER OF SIMPLICITY

In a time when sleek showers have replaced traditional bathtubs, the art of bathing for wellness has quietly faded. But therapeutic soaks remain one of the most effective, affordable ways to support the body's natural detox pathways—especially for those committed to long-term vitality.

During a period of intense healing, I returned to regular detox baths. The results were both restorative and transformative. I kept it simple with just two timeless ingredients:

- Baking Soda – Alkalizes the body, calms the skin, and leaves you feeling clean and renewed.
- Epsom Salt – Delivers a calming dose of magnesium while helping pull toxins and heavy metals through the skin.

That's it. No dyes. No synthetic fragrances. No bubble bath distractions. Just pure therapeutic soaking. The outcome? Better sleep, smoother skin, clearer thoughts, and a lightness in the body that's hard to describe—until you feel it yourself.

WHY I DON'T USE ESSENTIAL OILS

Essential oils have their place, but I've chosen to leave them out of my detox soaks. I've seen too many sensitivities and overreactions in people who overused them. For me, less is more. I'd rather use the whole herb—through teas or cooking—and stay close to nature. That's been my rule of thumb throughout this book.

BEAUTY FROM THE OUTSIDE IN

Your skin is a living, breathing detox organ—absorbing and eliminating constantly. When you support it with clean, purposeful ingredients like baking soda and Epsom salt, you're not just soothing the surface. You're helping your liver, your lymphatic system, your brain. You're feeding vitality from the outside in.

Let your home be your wellness sanctuary. Commit to small, consistent rituals that work with the body—not against it—and you'll see the reflection of that care in your skin, energy, and spirit.

Real minerals. Real relief. Real renewal.

Foot Soaks:
SWEAT IT OUT, SOAK IT IN

Real Detox That Starts from the Ground Up

When full-body baths aren't realistic, foot soaks are the ultimate home spa workaround. Simple, affordable, and surprisingly powerful, they offer deep detoxification from the ground up—without leaving your living room.

The skin on your feet is packed with sweat glands and nerve endings, making it one of the best exit points for toxins. Soaking your feet in warm, mineral-rich water opens your pores, encourages gentle sweating, and activates circulation—mimicking the benefits of a sauna session. Think of it as a detox drainage valve for your entire system.

MY SOAK SETUP: SIMPLE AND EFFECTIVE

Forget those tiny foot spa machines—they're messy, hard to clean, and overflow way too easily. I bought one, used it once, and never looked back.

Instead, we picked up BPA-free five-gallon buckets from Lowe's. Total game changers. They're deep, sturdy, and easy to clean. I fill mine with warm water, add a generous scoop of baking soda and Epsom salt, and set it on a towel in front of the couch.

Then we soak. And sweat. And detox.

For 30 minutes, my husband plays video games while I wind down with the dogs. It's our version of a home sauna—without the cost or clutter. The warmth triggers a light sweat, which helps push toxins out through the feet and promotes magnesium absorption throughout the body.

DIY FOOT SOAK RECIPE
Tools:
- BPA-free 5-gallon bucket
- Towel (for under bucket)
- Timer (optional)

Ingredients:
- Warm water (fill half bucket)
- 1/2 cup baking soda
- 3/4 cup Epsom salt

Instructions:
- 5 gallon bucket
- Add baking soda and Epsom salt
- Fill bucket with warm water (not too hot)
- Place bucket on towel in a comfortable area.
- Soak feet for 30 minutes while you relax, read, or watch a show

Tip: Do this 1-3 times a week for cumulative detox benefits.

The Benefits Are Real:
- Encourages sweating and toxin release
- Delivers magnesium to calm muscles and nerves
- Reduces foot and joint inflammation
- Improves circulation and lymphatic flow
- Supports better sleep, digestion, and energy

CONSISTENCY IS KEY

We soak twice a week. It's not about perfection—it's about steady, supportive routines that help your body reset. You'll feel lighter, more grounded, and noticeably less tense.

This isn't a trend. It's timeless.

Wellness doesn't have to be complicated.

The body knows how to heal—sometimes it just needs warm water, minerals, and a moment to let go.

"Glow begins at ground level—soak, sweat,
and let your radiance rise."

Castor Oil Packs:
DETOXING YOUR CORE AND
CALMING YOUR SYSTEM

Some remedies speak softly but carry deep, lasting power—and castor oil is one of them. The more I've used it, the more convinced I've become of its therapeutic value. It's simple, affordable, and incredibly effective for supporting sleep, digestion, detoxification, and full-body reset. A little goes a long way—and the results are anything but small.

This section shares how I've used castor oil in real life: not just as a throwback folk remedy, but as a consistent, restorative practice. Whether on the abdomen or the feet, castor oil has become one of the most versatile tools in my anti-aging wellness routine.

MY FIRST CASTOR OIL PACK EXPERIENCE

I began experimenting with castor oil packs during a particularly challenging time—trying to calm internal inflammation and find relief without prescriptions or guesswork. Like many of my favorite strategies, I pieced it together from my own research and a little creativity at home.

I started with cotton flannel cloths (I bought baby diaper cloths from Amazon), soaked them in castor oil, and placed them over my abdomen to cover the liver and digestive area.

We followed the traditional method:

- Place the oiled cloth directly on the skin
- Cover it with BPA-free plastic or wrap
- Add a towel layer
- Apply moist heat using a hot water bag or compress
- Lie back and relax for 30 minutes or more

After the first session, I experienced an unexpected and intense reaction—lightheadedness, disorientation, and a sudden sense of imbalance when trying to stand. It was a reminder that detoxification can sometimes be profound. I stayed calm, hydrated, and rested, and the symptoms subsided within an hour. The next session was smooth, uneventful, and incredibly relaxing. Often, the body just needs to adjust.

MY UPGRADED CASTOR OIL ROUTINE

Eventually, I traded in the thick, sticky castor oil for a lighter, more pure version from Heritage Store. It's still organic, but much smoother, easier to absorb, and more enjoyable to use.

These days, I follow a cleaner, simpler routine:

- Rub castor oil on core abdominal region
- Place a pre-moistened castor oil cloth on top
- Cover with BPA-free plastic
- Wrap everything in a soft, elastic 1 ft x 6 ft body wrap
- Skip the heat for a convenient, mess-free option
- Leave it on for an hour or more

This method feels like a tune-up for my entire midsection—stimulating circulation, supporting digestion, and potentially even helping eliminate parasites and other unwanted invaders. I believe it also aids the gut microbiome by clearing out harmful pathogens and refreshing my internal terrain.

FOOT APPLICATION FOR RESTORATIVE SLEEP

Also, I started using castor oil on the bottoms of my feet. It's gentler than a full pack but still deeply effective. I rub the oil in, slip on BPA-free plastic food bags, and secure them with a soft pair of socks. Then I relax for an hour or two, letting the oil do its quiet work.

This became one of my favorite wind-down rituals. Every time I do it, I sleep deeper, dream more vividly, and wake up feeling lighter. It's incredible how even external application can signal internal healing.

Tip: Always use a plastic barrier—castor oil is thick, and it can stain. If you get it on clothes or fabric, boiling water is your best bet for removal.

A FINAL WORD ON CASTOR OIL'S POWER

Castor oil has earned a permanent place in my wellness arsenal. Whether applied to the abdomen or the soles of the feet, its detoxifying, calming, and restorative effects are undeniable. It's affordable, easy to use, and endlessly versatile.

For the core materials, I keep my cloth folded and stored in a tray between uses and switch out the plastic bag each time for cleanliness. These small details make the process more sustainable and manageable long-term.

The castor oil pack isn't just a remedy—it's a ritual. It supports the organs at your body's core, flushes out stored waste, and contributes to that all-important sense of clarity, calm, and glow. Much like tuning up a car, this method gives your liver, gut, and immune system the refresh they deserve—so you can keep driving forward with energy, resilience, and youth on your side.

Reset your gut, refresh your glow—
one castor oil session at a time.

BAKING SODA BODY SPRAY: A REFRESHING ALKALINE BOOST

In a world overloaded with chemical fragrances and synthetic personal care products, I've learned to take a gentler, more intentional approach. Over time, I developed a sensitivity to perfumes and scented body sprays—something that only increased with age and toxic buildup. What once felt "fresh" quickly became irritating and overwhelming to my senses.

So I made my own solution: a simple, natural baking soda body spray. No fragrance, no fluff—just a clean, cooling mist that helps refresh, rebalance, and restore your skin's natural calm.

THE POWER OF SIMPLICITY: A MIST WITH A PURPOSE

This spray was a natural evolution of my baking soda habits. I was already using it in foot soaks and toenail care, so creating a body mist felt like the next logical step. Especially for those moments when you want to feel clean and reset—without needing to take a full shower.

Baking soda is naturally alkaline, making it an excellent ally for balancing skin pH, calming inflammation, and neutralizing surface-level pathogens. It has a soothing, grounding effect—especially after a hot shower when my arms used to turn red and reactive. A few spritzes of the mist and the irritation would fade almost immediately.

WAYS I USE IT:
- Sprayed across arms, legs, back—anywhere skin feels warm or flushed
- Directly on the feet after a long day

- On sensitive patches of skin that feel itchy, dry, or irritated
- As a midday refresh when I don't feel like showering again

This simple formula leaves me feeling clean and uplifted—without the chemical fog of artificial fragrance. It's a clear example of how powerful everyday ingredients can be when we lean into natural self-care instead of synthetic solutions.

WHY IT WORKS
- Alkalizes the skin to support a balanced pH
- Soothes inflammation and redness after bathing
- Naturally deodorizes without synthetic fragrances
- Cleanses and refreshes when you don't have time to shower
- Antimicrobial benefits help support healthy skin flora

No perfumes. No toxins.
Just clarity, calm, and confidence—

"Simplicity isn't boring—it's healing."
Sometimes the most powerful skin treatments come from your pantry, not a product line.

WHY EXTERNAL DETOX MATTERS
Your skin isn't just a surface—it's a detox organ. Through practices like foot soaks, castor oil packs, and baking soda body sprays, you're not just pampering yourself. You're activating natural cleansing systems that support lymphatic drainage, reduce inflammation, and promote radiant skin.
These rituals:
- Calm the nervous system
- Stimulate circulation
- Encourage restful sleep
- Support digestive balance

- Improve skin texture
- Boost full-body vitality

RESTORATIVE RITUALS
FOR LIFELONG RADIANCE

True wellness isn't confined to what we eat or the supplements we take—it's a full-body experience, and the skin is a vital part of that story. These home spa rituals—foot soaks, castor oil packs, and baking soda body sprays—aren't indulgences. They're intentional, restorative therapies that help the body detoxify, reset, and renew.

When we embrace simple, grounding practices, we support our body's natural rhythm to heal and strengthen. We encourage better sleep, improve skin texture, support digestion, balance our inner environment, and ultimately extend our vitality and youthfulness.

The beauty of these routines is that they're real. They don't require memberships or expensive products—just commitment, awareness, and a willingness to listen to your body.

Consistency over perfection. Natural over synthetic. Inner healing that radiates outward.

That's the formula for aging well and living fully.

True detoxification is a lifestyle, not a weekend cleanse.

Real strategies. Real results. Real rejuvenation.

CHAPTER 10

RADIATION

THE INVISIBLE AGITATOR

"It's the way of the world."

That's what people say—and they're not wrong.

Radiation is everywhere now. It's built into our lives—from the sun above to the phones in our hands, from smart meters to Wi-Fi routers. We can't fully escape it, but we can stop pretending it doesn't matter.

I'm not writing this from a bunker in the woods. I'm writing it on a laptop, connected to Wi-Fi, in a world running on devices and screens. And yes, even writing this book is likely radiating me. But that's not the point. The point is awareness. The point is action.

We don't need fear—we need strategy. The goal isn't to unplug from society, but to make smarter choices where we can. Protect the body. Reduce exposure. Heal what gets thrown off course. Whether it's walking barefoot to ground yourself, switching off devices at night, or rethinking where your head rests while you sleep—these decisions matter. They add up.

Radiation might be the way of the world, but so is resilience. And in this chapter, we'll look at real, practical ways to protect your health, slow aging, and feel better in a high-frequency world.

MICROWAVE COOKING

A Convenient Mistake That Costs Too Much

Back in the 1980s, the microwave was the gold standard of convenience. Everyone had one. Everyone used it. Frozen dinners, hot water, leftover pizza — you name it. I was no different. As a kid and even into my twenties, I used the microwave constantly. It was just what people did.

But I started noticing something. Food didn't taste right. It was soggy, rubbery, lifeless. Nothing that came out of a microwave had that real, vibrant energy food is supposed to give. Still, I kept using it now and then — until I saw the plant test.

THE WAKE-UP CALL: A SIMPLE EXPERIMENT

I saw a video of a simple experiment:

A young girl ran a home science project. Two plants. One watered with regular water, the other with water that had been microwaved. The plant fed microwaved water wilted and died. The other one thrived. That was it for me. If microwaved water can kill a plant, what's it doing to our food — and our bodies?

That was the turning point. I stopped cooking food in the microwave altogether.

REAL FOOD, REAL HEAT, REAL FLAVOR

We started making everything on the stove or in the oven. And it made a difference. Real cooking brought food back to life. The flavor was richer. The texture made sense. It felt nourishing again. Even heating leftovers on the stovetop or in the oven felt like an upgrade.

We still used the microwave for heating up plates — until the repair guy said that could actually break the unit. Plates don't absorb radiation the way food does, so it was frying the inside of the machine. That was all I needed to hear. Since then, we've repurposed it as a kitchen timer and light source, opting to warm plates in the oven or on the stovetop.

DINING OUT? NOT MUCH.

We eat out maybe five times a year. And there's a reason. I've worked in restaurants. I know how food is prepared behind the scenes. Microwaves are everywhere. From sauces to proteins, it's the quick-fix method to speed up service. But quick doesn't mean quality. Why would I pay extra to eat radiated food that tastes worse and digests poorly? I'd rather stay home and cook a real meal with real ingredients.

WHY IT MATTERS FOR ANTI-AGING

Microwaves don't just heat food — they change it. The structure. The texture. The nutrient profile. All altered. Some studies even show that microwaving processed meats can lead to harmful byproducts linked to inflammation and heart disease.

In a world already overloaded with toxins and stress, why add another invisible burden to your body? This is about more than taste — it's about protecting your energy, your cells, and your youth.

WHAT I DO INSTEAD

I warm plates in the oven or set them on the stove while I cook. Leftovers go in a pan or in the oven— never the microwave. It takes more time, but your body knows the difference. Better digestion. Better taste. Better results.

In the end, it's not just about avoiding radiation. It's about giving your body the fuel it deserves. When you prepare food with care, your body rewards you. You feel younger. Stronger. More grounded.

And once you break free from the microwave habit, you won't want to go back.

Real heat. Real flavor. Real health.

Why I Don't Microwave:
- It alters the texture and flavor of food
- Radiation exposure—even minimal—is cumulative

- Heating plastics can leach toxins into your food
- It's not how our grandparents cooked—and they aged better
- Cooking from scratch just tastes better and feels better

Don't Radiate. Rejuvenate.
Return to Real Cooking.

GROUNDING:
A PRACTICAL DEFENSE AGAINST DAILY RADIATION

Simple adjustments that protect your health—and your peace of mind

When we installed solar panels, I wasn't thinking about radiation. I just wanted to save on electricity. But once the panels were up, people started commenting—mocking, even—that I was now living under a radiation field. It caught me off guard. Was this really a problem?

Being a health-minded person, I wasn't going to ignore it. I ordered an EMF reader and decided to check for myself.

THE EYE-OPENING REALITY OF EMF EXPOSURE
I started in the room directly under the solar panels. Surprisingly, no high readings there. But once I began scanning electronics and especially the walls, things got interesting fast.

The alarm clock next to the bed lit up the EMF reader like a siren. I'd been sleeping inches from it for years. The TV across the room wasn't much better. Even more shocking? Radiation hotspots where outlets were—including spots where the outlet was actually on the other side of the wall. One of the highest EMF zones was exactly where my head had been resting each night.

We moved the bed to a different wall that same day. The alarm clock now sits on a table across the room. The TV is farther away. Small changes—big relief.

GROUNDING TOOLS I ACTUALLY USE

After seeing the numbers firsthand, I started researching how to offset this exposure. We got a cover for our Wi-Fi router. That made a noticeable difference. The keyboard and computer still give off a strong signal, but now I use a grounding mat under the mouse pad. I ordered from the original creators at Earthing.com—they even sent me a copy of their book. It was worth reading.

Now we also have grounding pillowcases, sheets, and even extras for the dogs. When I use a laptop or gaming controller, I place them over one of the grounding cases. The dogs seem to gravitate to them too—proof enough for me.

OTHER HIDDEN RADIATION SOURCES

Some of the worst offenders were things I used daily:

- My light-up makeup mirror: off-the-charts radiation. I still use it, but only unplugged.
- Hair dryer: high EMF levels. I stand on a grounding mat while using it now.
- Phone charger: I never plug it in by the bed anymore. Four feet away minimum.

None of this is about fear—it's about calling it like it is. Radiation exposure adds up, and your body feels it: the headaches, the fog, the slow drag on your energy. But when you cut it down? You think faster. Sleep harder. Look better. These grounding tools aren't perfect—but they work. And in a world full of invisible stressors, staying sharp is the real power move—one that shows up in your skin, your energy, and how young you really feel.

Guard exposure. Ground your body. Glow with vitality.

Everyday Defense:
GEAR THAT PROTECTS

In a world where tech follows us everywhere, radiation is always just inches away—from our hands, pockets, and bedsides. While we can't eliminate our devices, we can be smart about how we interact with them. Protective gear isn't paranoia—it's prevention. If you're going to carry it, touch it, and sleep near it, make it as safe as possible.

SMART SHIELDS: PRACTICAL EMF PROTECTION

We all use cell phones and portable devices, so it only makes sense to protect ourselves where we can. There are plenty of companies offering shielding products, but the brand I chose was Safe Sleeve. These phone cases are specifically designed to block radiation from reaching your body.

Of course, I didn't just take their word for it. I grabbed my EMF reader and ran the test myself.

I first measured the phone's radiation without the case. As expected, the readings were high—especially when making a call. Then, I closed the case and tested again while still on the call. The drop was immediate and significant. That sealed the deal for me. Knowing the case actively reduced exposure while I was holding the phone to my head made a huge difference. Since the shielded flap stays between your face and the device during use, you're not absorbing that excess radiation every time you talk.

For anyone who carries their phone in a pocket—especially men who don't use bags—this kind of protective case is a must. Radiation exposure adds up over time, and small steps like this matter.

In a world that's already too connected and overexposed, I love knowing I'm doing something, however small, to cut down on what my body has to endure. It's these real-life choices that add up to long-term resilience, youthfulness, and peace of mind.

LESS EXPOSURE. MORE RADIANCE.

We may not be able to eliminate radiation from modern life, but we can choose how we interact with it. From microwaves and routers to chargers and cell phones, the exposure is constant—but it doesn't have to be careless. Small shifts add up. Rearranging your bedroom, grounding your body, shielding your devices—these aren't extremes. They're strategies. We protect our skin from sun damage; why not protect our nervous system from EMFs?

This chapter isn't about panic—it's about power. Real health isn't passive. It's deliberate. When you take steps to reduce radiation exposure, you're preserving energy, supporting your cells, and strengthening your body's resilience.

And in a world that's wired, taking action —even a little—can be one of the most anti-aging decisions you make.

Block the radiation. Shield your body.
Protect your future.

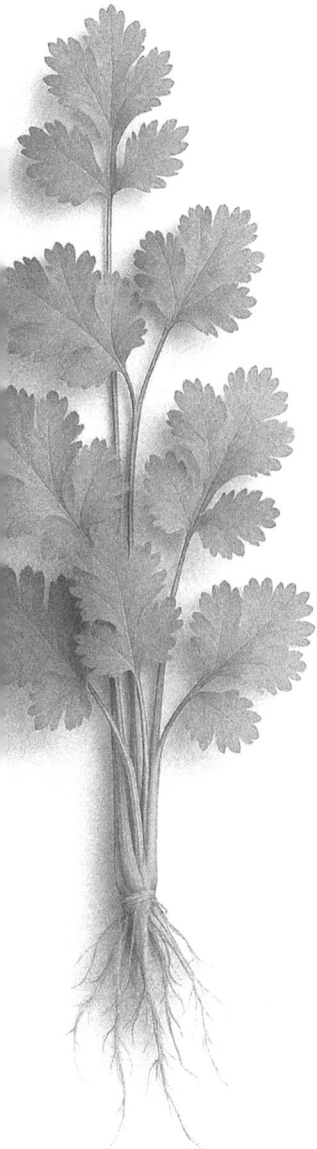

PART 4

A SOUND
MIND

CHAPTER 11

A SOUND MIND

RECLAIMING YOUR MENTAL EDGE

Clear Thinking, Grounded Living, and the Strength to Stay Sharp

Youth isn't just about what you see in the mirror—it's about how you think, how you feel, and how your mind processes the world around you. A sound mind is one of the most valuable anti-aging assets we have. It affects everything: decision-making, memory, mood, and our capacity to live with peace and purpose.

But mental clarity doesn't exist in isolation. It's deeply tied to physical health. Nutrient deficiencies, toxic buildup, heavy metals, and even overuse of certain supplements can cloud the mind. The good news? These are obstacles you can do something about. When you tune in to your body's signals and become an active participant in your own well-being, everything begins to shift.

As kids, most of us never thought twice about mental clarity. We absorbed life as it came—playfully, instinctively. But as we age, we start to recognize the power of the mind as both a tool and a reflection. And the more we understand it, the more we can shape its direction. You are not a prisoner to foggy thinking, low energy, or emotional instability. You are capable of clarity.

This chapter explores the many threads that support a sound mind— physical detox strategies, spiritual alignment, nutritional awareness, stress reduction, and mental stimulation. We'll talk about real, daily choices that nourish the brain and protect it from decline:

- ▸ Avoiding toxic inputs
- ▸ Living honestly and without internal conflict
- ▸ Reducing the influence of alcohol, drugs, and overstimulation
- ▸ Cultivating active learning and curiosity
- ▸ And most importantly, inviting God into the process—for He is the one who gives us a spirit-not of fear, but of power, love, and a sound mind.

A detoxed mind and a clear head free you to fully engage with life—awake, present, and alive.

CLEARING THE MIND:
WHEN IT'S MORE THAN JUST MENTAL

Sometimes what we call "mental" has physical roots. I learned this firsthand.

After battling a period of neuritis, my view of mental wellness shifted entirely. That experience gave me a deeper level of compassion for anyone dealing with unexplained brain fog, anxiety, or that uneasy sense that something just feels off. It also taught me that real healing often starts with asking the harder question: What's really going on beneath the surface?

ANXIETY ISN'T ALWAYS JUST ANXIETY
These days, "anxiety" has become a catch-all. But sometimes it's not a mood disorder—it's a symptom. A deeper imbalance. For me, anxiety wasn't just in my head—it was in my body. And it was pointing to something bigger.

Heavy metals. Inflammation. Hormonal shifts. Toxin buildup. All of these can impact brain function and emotional regulation. If something inside is misfiring, it's no wonder the mind starts to feel scrambled.

ALUMINUM: THE HIDDEN OFFENDER

One of the first things I cleaned up was aluminum exposure. It's a known neurotoxin, and it's everywhere—from deodorants to cookware to canned food.

Here's what I implement:

▸ Deodorant: I use a natural salt stick—completely aluminum-free.
▸ Cookware: I use cast iron and stainless steel. For baking, I use glass or ceramic.
▸ Canned foods: If you have to buy them, find cans with BPA liner. We focus on fresh, frozen, or glass-packed instead.

These small shifts matter. Even invisible toxins can cause real disruption.

SUPPORT FOR HEAVY METAL DETOX

I also leaned on natural supports like:

▸ Iodine – known to displace halogens and support thyroid and detox.
▸ Cilantro – a gentle chelator that helps pull metals from the body.

These are powerful allies to implement.

THE OXALATE WILDCARD

Oxalates are another overlooked trigger. These plant compounds build up in the body and can cause inflammation, joint pain, even mental fog. I didn't realize how much I was consuming until I looked into it—spinach, almonds, beets, sweet potatoes. All healthy foods... or so I thought.

I tried reducing high-oxalate foods for a while and noticed improvements. That's the beauty of experimenting. You never know what might be weighing you down until you lighten the load.

DON'T FORGET TO SWEAT

Sweating is an ancient form of detox. It's free, primal, and powerful.

- Epsom salt baths
- Foot soaks
- Sun exposure
- Workout sessions that make you sweat

If your pores aren't pushing out toxins, those toxins stay in. Circulation improves. The mind feels clearer. Everything flows better when you sweat.

THE GAME CHANGER:
MSM AND DIATOMACEOUS EARTH

After three years of constant anxiety and not feeling like myself, also dealing with cystitis for over a year, I had all but run out of hope. I'd tried every herb, every supplement—always natural, always clean. Nothing worked. Then came the turning point.

I was standing in line at Herbally Grounded, my local health shop. I picked up two things: MSM and diatomaceous earth. I had no grand plan. I just had a feeling. And that feeling turned into freedom.

These are the only two supplements that truly reset my brain and body. After years of searching, I finally found what worked.

- Diatomaceous Earth: 1 tablespoon, up to 3x daily at first, now 1x for maintenance. Rich in silica, it helps clear pathogens and supports detox.
- MSM (Sulfur): Up to 8,000 mg daily, spread out. Supports collagen, hormones, skin, and—most notably for me—mental clarity.

And just like that... everything changed.

Within days, the anxiety began to lift. My body recalibrated. My mind felt like mine again. The cystitis disappeared. The fog cleared. I felt like I was back.

MSM became my personal favorite to assist in mental clarity. It's a sulfur compound that is a prime component in all of our cells effecting proteins, collagen, keratin, hormones, and enzymes.

NEVER GIVE UP

I don't say this lightly: if something isn't right in your body or mind, don't stop searching. The solution might be something you haven't tried yet. One new product. One detox ritual. One shift in thinking.

I share this not as a cure—but as a path. And sometimes, the right path changes everything.

"Mental fog isn't your new normal.
Clarity is still possible—just detox and don't give up."

Too Much of a Good Thing:
THE VITAMIN D WAKE-UP CALL

Not every supplement is as harmless as it seems—especially when taken long term and at high doses. This is one story I'll never forget.

A few years back, my doctor recommended I take 2,000 IU of vitamin D daily to correct low levels. That seemed reasonable. But then came the suggestions from friends and wellness circles—"10,000 IU a day is where the real results are." It was the same price, and more sounded better. So, we made the jump.

Everything seemed fine for a few years… until it wasn't.

THE DAY OUR BRAINS GLITCHED

In 2017, the same year I developed neuritis, I started noticing something strange. In large stores—especially ones with lots of bright lights and stocked shelves—my brain couldn't keep up. It was as if the information was coming in too fast for my visual system to process. I'd walk into a store and feel completely overwhelmed, like my brain was flickering between "on" and "off."

One day, my husband and I walked into Lowe's, and right away I started feeling that visual overload again. But then—confirmation. My husband blurted out, "What the heck is this!" He was seeing and feeling it too. I was so relieved. "You can see it?" I asked. He could. We both stood there stunned.

We hadn't been taking many supplements at the time—mainly vitamins. So I started researching every ingredient in our daily regimen. That's when I came across a reference linking high-dose vitamin D with cognitive disruption, particularly in how the brain processes spatial and visual data. It was subtle, but real.

THE FIX WAS SIMPLE

We cut our dose back to 1,000 IU daily. And that bizarre brain static disappeared. Gone. Neither of us has experienced it since.

TRACK WHAT YOU TAKE

It was a lesson I won't forget: more isn't always better. Supplements are powerful. They can support or sabotage depending on how they're used. Since then, I've made journaling part of my routine—tracking what I take, how I feel, and any changes that surface.

Know your body. Watch for patterns. And when in doubt—scale back and observe. Sometimes less is exactly what your brain needs to think clearly and age wisely.

"Natural doesn't mean harmless—
know your body, know your dose."

DON'T DO DRUGS:
A CLEAR MIND IS WORTH MORE

The Illusion of Relief

It shouldn't come as a surprise—drugs come with consequences. Whether they're legal, illegal, or prescription, they affect your health, your energy, and your brain. There's this illusion that they fix things. But they don't fix anything. At best, they offer a temporary patch. At worst, they create new problems, often worse than the one you started with.

I'm not saying there's never a place for medication. But we've gone off the rails as a culture. Popping a pill for every issue has become the norm—and that's dangerous. Many of these drugs are known to dull cognition, alter mood, and even contribute to dementia over time.

DRUGS AND THE BRAIN

Pharmaceuticals may seem helpful in the short term, but they can come with long-term effects that sabotage your mental clarity. That includes everything from brain fog and fatigue to emotional numbness and memory loss. Some prescription drugs are even linked to changes in the structure of the brain.

For a society so concerned with looking young, we're awfully quick to trade away our mental youth.

FALSE COMFORT, REAL DAMAGE

There's always a cost. And that cost is rarely printed clearly on the label. You might not feel the effects right away—but over time, your body knows. Your liver, your hormones, your neurotransmitters—they're all paying the price.

The anti-aging lifestyle isn't about numbing what we feel. It's about healing from the inside out. That includes emotional discomfort, stress, and pain. Masking those things doesn't make them disappear. It just pushes the problem further down the line.

REAL HEALING OVER QUICK FIXES

I've known people who went the quick-fix route. And I've seen the toll it takes—physically, mentally, and emotionally. I'm not interested in that path. And I don't want that for you, either.

The better strategy? Stay clean. Stay clear. Take the time to dig deeper. The real solution is almost always simpler than we think—natural tools, consistent routines, and honest reflection. Real peace doesn't come in a pill bottle. It comes from clarity, purpose, and health that's built day by day.

Stay sharp. Stay clean. Stay real.

Alcohol:
A CULTURALLY ACCEPTED TOXIN

It's no secret that drinking is a social norm. In fact, it's often celebrated. But what rarely gets mentioned is the lasting toll it takes on the brain—especially when consumed over the long haul.

THE SILENT DAMAGE TO THE BRAIN

Alcohol-Related Brain Damage (ARBD) is very real—and very overlooked. Years of regular drinking can destroy the very nerve cells you need to think clearly, move smoothly, and function as your best self. If we're striving for vibrancy, clarity, and a sound mind into our later years, reducing or eliminating alcohol should be near the top of the list.

OUR JOURNEY: FROM CASUAL DRINKERS TO NONE AT ALL

Before 2017, alcohol was still part of our lifestyle. Like most people, we had our drinks. Beer. Wine. Occasional liquor.

When we became Christians in 2001, we felt the desire to quit—multiple times, in fact. But addiction has its grip. It's not just about willpower; it's about rewiring the mind and removing the emotional hooks. Even as we told ourselves things like, "Wine is good for the heart," we knew deep down we wanted a change.

THE DAY IT ALL SHIFTED
And then one day, it happened. A deep conviction settled in—and this time, it stuck. God gave us the strength to walk away from it completely. That moment was life-changing. My husband and I both quit, and we've never looked back.

Quitting wasn't easy, but it was absolutely worth it. Mental clarity, deeper sleep, emotional stability, and a lighter, more energized body—all the things we aim for in anti-aging came into sharper focus once alcohol was out of the picture.

IF YOU'RE STRUGGLING TO QUIT
Don't give up. We tried for sixteen years. We'd "take breaks" and tell ourselves it wasn't that bad. But once we finally let it go, everything improved. My husband always jokes, "After the first two years, it's all downhill." Now we laugh about it—but we're also deeply grateful.

MENTAL DETOX:
WHAT WE DO TO OURSELVES

Self-Induced Stress and the Power of Integrity

After addressing the physical contributors to brain fog and mental imbalance, we also have to take responsibility for the mental clutter we sometimes create ourselves. Not every burden comes from outside. Some of the heaviest weights are self-inflicted—and that's actually good news. It means we have the power to stop carrying them.

THE QUIET STRESS OF POOR CHOICES
There are thought patterns and daily decisions that generate stress in ways we don't always notice at first. Maybe it's guilt from something we

said. Or something we're hiding. Maybe we're consuming content that feels "normal" in the moment but subtly pollutes the mind. The result? Internal chaos. Emotional drain. Accelerated aging.

This kind of stress isn't always dramatic. It's quiet and cumulative. But it ages you all the same.

INTEGRITY IS ANTI-AGING

Living with honesty is one of the most underrated health strategies there is. Are you being truthful with others—and yourself? Are you white-lying your way through uncomfortable moments, thinking it won't matter?

It matters.

Guilt ages you. So does living out of alignment with what you know to be good. A clean conscience is more powerful than a green smoothie. It clears your mind, lifts your mood, and boosts vitality from within. Integrity produces peace—and peace is energizing.

MONITOR THE INPUTS

What we feed our minds is just as important as what we feed our bodies. Choose entertainment and education that uplifts or enlightens. Avoid media that degrades your spirit. Keep your thoughts pure and focused. When your mind isn't distracted by garbage, it has the space to grow sharper, calmer, and more creative.

THIS ISN'T ABOUT PERFECTION

It's about alignment. The goal isn't to be flawless—it's to live in such a way that your daily actions match your deepest values. When they do, the tension lifts. The brain feels lighter. The mind clears. And you start to feel steady and clear—like your best self has finally caught up to you.

Mental detox isn't just about removing external toxins. It's also about clearing internal conflict. And the simplest way to start is by making choices you can stand behind—with no regrets and no residue.

Real choices. Real integrity. Real peace of mind

STAY CURIOUS:
LEARNING AS A LIFELONG STRATEGY FOR YOUTHFUL VITALITY

One of the most powerful ways to keep your mind sharp and spirit youthful is to keep learning. Curiosity is anti-aging. Not in theory—literally. When you learn something new, your brain forms new neural pathways, keeps your memory mechanisms active, and encourages plasticity, which helps slow cognitive decline. I truly believe curiosity is a key pillar of a vibrant life. It keeps us from going stale, stuck, or sluggish.

For me, learning isn't just about books or formal courses. It's about staying mentally engaged. I ask questions. I watch how people do things. I get interested in things I've never tried before. That might mean learning about ancient remedies, trying a new form of exercise, experimenting with homemade recipes, or even researching a topic just because it lights a spark in me. That spark is youth.

When we were kids, we were constantly asking why. That same habit still works as we age. The brain is built to grow—but only if we keep feeding it. And the best food for the brain isn't just fat or minerals (though I'm a fan of those, too). It's newness. New thoughts. New ideas. New challenges. We can stretch our cognitive muscles every day by simply staying interested.

TRY THIS

Pick a subject you've always been curious about—even if it seems unrelated to health. Bees? Carpentry? Natural dyes? Brain waves? Learn something about it this week. Not for performance. Just for pleasure. This habit alone can bring back a fire you didn't know you were missing. Curiosity is free. It's deeply nourishing. And it's available for life.

The moment you stop learning
is the moment you start aging.

BRAIN-BOOSTING CURIOSITY STARTERS

Keep your mind energized with just a few minutes a day:

- ‣ Learn a word in another language.
- ‣ Watch a short doc on something random—volcanoes, beekeeping, how violins are made.
- ‣ Ask "why?" about something you do every day—then look it up.
- ‣ Try a new route when walking or driving.
- ‣ Switch hands while brushing teeth or writing a list—activate different brain areas.
- ‣ Listen to a podcast that's way outside your normal zone.
- ‣ Pick up a book from a section you never browse.

Keep stretching. The more you explore, the more alive your mind stays.

New thoughts. New growth. Timeless mind.

God-Given Clarity:
A SOUND MIND AS THE FOUNDATION OF HEALTH

Faith Isn't Separate from Health—It's the Starting Point

Just like our bodies need clean food and natural supplements, our minds need truth, stability, and alignment. Cognitive clarity is essential for long-term vitality. A well-functioning brain helps us make better choices, stay motivated, and carry peace throughout the day. And the deepest source of that clarity? It comes from God.

He didn't just design the body to heal—He designed the mind to be renewed. Scripture reminds us that we aren't left to wander in mental fog or emotional imbalance. Through faith, we're offered a sound mind—stable, empowered, and capable of discerning truth in a noisy world.

We prioritize gut health, clear skin, and deep sleep—but the real anti-aging foundation begins in the mind. And it's strengthened when you trust the One who created it.

POWER, LOVE, AND A SOUND MIND
God's Word makes it clear:

> *"For God hath not given us the spirit of fear; but of*
> *power, and of love, and of a sound mind."*
> *— 2 Timothy 1:7 (KJV)*

This verse isn't just encouragement—it's a blueprint. When we're grounded in faith, fear loses its grip. Mental clarity soars. We step into confidence, discernment, and peace. And in that space, the mind becomes sharp, alert, and calm—not anxious, distracted, or defeated.

WISDOM IS HEALTH
Proverbs and James echo the same theme: true wisdom is available, and it's deeply connected to health.

"He layeth up sound wisdom for the righteous: he is a buckler to them that walk uprightly." — Proverbs 2:7

"If any of you lack wisdom, let him ask of God… and it shall be given him." — James 1:5

Walking in wisdom is a protection—it keeps our choices clean, our emotions steady, and our days productive. And if clarity ever feels out of reach, we can simply ask. That's the beauty of it.

LONGEVITY BEGINS IN THE MIND
Having a sound mind isn't just spiritual—it's biological. Clear thinking reduces stress, supports hormonal balance, sharpens memory, and keeps you motivated to stay healthy. When your thoughts are aligned with truth, your body follows suit. You sleep better. You digest better. You age better.

"A sound heart is the life of the flesh…"
— Proverbs 14:30

That's what we're after: life-giving practices that preserve our energy, protect our mental space, and help us age with grace.

LET THIS BE YOUR ANCHOR

A sound mind is more than a goal—it's a gift. Fill your thoughts with truth. Ask for wisdom. Walk uprightly. Speak sound words. And let your faith become the foundation for mental strength that sustains your health for decades to come.

2 Timothy 1:13 Hold fast the form of sound words, which thou hast heard of me, in faith and love which is in Christ Jesus. (KJV)

GOD'S WISDOM. MENTAL STRENGTH. LASTING VITALITY.

In the pursuit of real health, we can't ignore the mind. A strong, sound mind doesn't just help us think clearly—it helps us live clearly. Our choices become sharper. Our emotions steadier. Our bodies lighter. And when that clarity is rooted in God's wisdom, the strength we build isn't just mental—it's spiritual, lasting, and deeply life-giving.

God has not left us guessing. He gives us clear instruction, calming truth, and the power to walk in love, not fear. A sound mind is His gift—and when we live in alignment with that design, it shows. In our energy. In our decisions. In our joy.

This is where anti-aging really begins—not just with creams, supplements, or routines, but with wisdom from above, a detoxed brain, and the peace of knowing you're living in truth. Let that be the foundation for a life that doesn't just last—but thrives.

"Health starts in the mind, and the healthiest minds are rooted in truth."

CONCLUSION

OWN YOUR YOUTHFULNESS. LIVE IT FULLY.

This isn't the end—it's the start of something stronger.

You now have a full toolkit of real-life strategies to protect your energy, restore your glow, and sharpen your mind. These aren't trendy tips—they're time-tested truths. From your first bite of breakfast to your final evening wind-down, everything you do builds the life you're living tomorrow. You get to choose how that looks.

You've learned how to make food work for you—whole, unprocessed, and clean. You've seen how homemade beats packaged, every time. You've taken control of your meals, your supplements, your skincare, your space. You've simplified to amplify.

Every single strategy in this book points back to one thing: power.

Power to rebuild.
Power to detox.
Power to glow.
Power to own your health.

You're not following a plan. You're living with purpose. The kind that says, I'm not settling for sluggishness, fog, or slow decline. Not anymore.

You've got momentum now. Not frantic, hype-fueled momentum—but deep, steady, unstoppable momentum. The kind that comes from clean habits, clear thinking, and confidence in what you're doing.

And most importantly—you're not doing this alone.

God gave you a sound mind. He designed your body to thrive. When you clear the path, when you remove the interference, He fills you with clarity, strength, and direction. That's when healing happens. That's when youth is restored. That's when your life regains its spark.

So show up fully. Eat well. Move freely. Detox regularly. Think sharply.

Refuse to numb out. Refuse to slow down. Refuse to accept a version of life that's less than what was meant for you.

You were designed for vitality.

You were built to radiate.

Now go live it.

Vibrant body. Clear mind. Unstoppable life.

May your strength stay steady,
your body stay sharp,
and your mind stay sound.
Live boldly. Think clearly.
You were made to radiate.

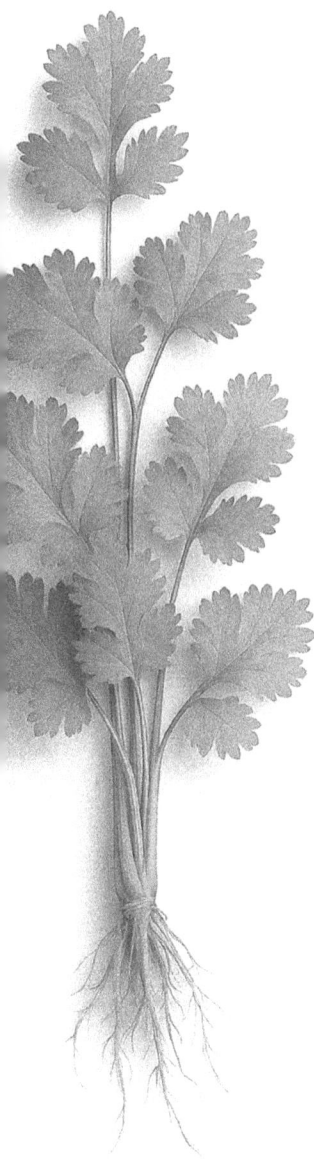

RECIPES

REAL LIFE RECIPES: FUEL FOR VIBRANT LIVING

T hese aren't just recipes—they're strategies. Every meal, every sip, every homemade mix in this section reflects the same health philosophy woven through this book: real ingredients, no nonsense, full impact. I make these myself. They're quick, clean, and rooted in purpose— from nourishing your cells to supporting detox, skin health, digestion, and clarity.

This is how I eat, drink, and thrive in real life. And now, it's yours to try too.

CORN SPOON BREAD

A rich, old-school comfort bake—simple, warm, and naturally satisfying.

INGREDIENTS:
- 1 quart whole milk
- ½ cup water
- 1 cup yellow corn flour
- 1 cup yellow cornmeal
- 4 eggs, separated
- 4 tablespoons melted butter
- 1½ teaspoons salt
- ½ teaspoon black pepper

DIRECTIONS:
1. Preheat oven to 375°F.
2. In a saucepan, bring milk and water to a gentle boil.
3. Stir in cornmeal, salt, and pepper.
4. Remove from heat. Stir in egg yolks and melted butter.
5. In a separate bowl, beat egg whites until stiff peaks form.
6. Gently fold beaten egg whites into the corn mixture.
7. Pour into a buttered 9x12 baking dish.
8. Bake for 45 minutes until golden, puffed, and set.

REAL LIFE TIP:
After cooling, slice into individual servings and wrap in sandwich bags. Place them all in a gallon-size freezer bag for easy storage. When ready to enjoy, reheat in the oven at 300°F for about 30 minutes. Perfect texture, no sogginess, no microwave needed.

REAL COLESLAW

Clean crunch. No mayo. Just raw, vibrant ingredients that refresh and support digestion.

INGREDIENTS:
- 1 cup chopped red cabbage
- 1 cup chopped green cabbage
- 2½ tablespoons apple cider vinegar
- 2½ tablespoons extra virgin organic olive oil
- ¼ teaspoon Celtic sea salt
- ¼ teaspoon organic black pepper or white pepper
- ¼ teaspoon cayenne pepper
- 1 tablespoon raw honey

DIRECTIONS:
1. Combine all ingredients in a large bowl and toss until well coated.
2. Cover and chill in the fridge for at least 1 day or overnight.
3. Stir before serving. The flavors intensify beautifully as it sits.

REAL LIFE TIP:
This slaw gets better with time. It's not just a side—it's a raw, cleansing addition to any meal. Great with grilled meats or as a crunchy topper for soups and stews.

BAKED FRENCH FRIES

A clean, crispy classic—no fryer, no weird oils. Just real potatoes done right.

INGREDIENTS:
- 1 Idaho potato per person (peeled or unpeeled)
- Extra virgin olive oil
- Celtic sea salt

DIRECTIONS:
1. Preheat oven to 425°F.
2. Push each potato through a potato press or cut into thin, even slices.
3. Soak slices in a bowl of cold water for 5 minutes.
4. Drain and pat completely dry with paper towels.
5. Toss in a bowl with olive oil and salt.
6. Spread evenly on a baking sheet.
7. Bake for 40 minutes, flipping halfway through, until golden and crisp on the edges.

REAL LIFE TIP:
These fries are best fresh from the oven. Serve with clean ketchup or homemade dipping sauce.

DOG CHICKEN

Simple, real food for your four-legged companions—because they deserve clean fuel too.

INGREDIENTS:
- 10–15 pounds organic boneless, skinless chicken thighs
- Celtic sea salt and black pepper (optional, light seasoning)

DIRECTIONS:
1. Preheat oven to 350°F.
2. Arrange chicken thighs on baking trays in a single layer.
3. Lightly season with salt and pepper (optional—omit for extra-sensitive dogs).
4. Bake for 25 minutes.
5. Flip each piece, then bake another 25 minutes until fully cooked.
6. Let cool, then cut into bite-sized cubes.
7. Portion about ½ cup into individual sandwich bags.
8. Store all sandwich bags in a large freezer bag.
9. Defrost one bag in the fridge overnight before serving.

REAL LIFE TIP:
Your pets thrive on whole, cooked meats just like we do. Keeping pre-portioned meals in the freezer makes clean feeding easy—and gives you peace of mind knowing they're eating real food, not fillers.

PECAN SANDIES

Buttery, nutty, melt-in-your-mouth cookies made with clean ingredients and none of the store-bought additives.

INGREDIENTS:
- ½ cup organic sugar
- 2 sticks (1 cup) organic butter, softened
- 2½ cups all-purpose flour
- ⅓ cup finely chopped pecans
- 1 teaspoon vanilla extract

DIRECTIONS:
1. In a large bowl, cream softened butter with sugar until smooth.
2. Add vanilla and mix well.
3. Gradually add flour, mixing until dough begins to form.
4. Stir in chopped pecans.
5. Divide dough into two 12-inch logs. Wrap and chill for 1 hour.
6. Preheat oven to 325°F. Line baking sheets with parchment paper.
7. Slice chilled dough into ¼-inch rounds and place on prepared sheets.
8. Bake for 18–20 minutes until lightly golden around the edges.

REAL LIFE TIP:
These store beautifully. Once cooled, store in air tight bag in freezer. A perfect little treat when you want something sweet without all the preservatives.

CHOCOLATE MACADAMIA NUT SCONES

Lightly sweet, buttery, and balanced with healthy fats from macadamias—finished with a drizzle of dark chocolate.

INGREDIENTS:

- 2¼ cups organic flour
- ¼ cup organic sugar
- 1 tablespoon baking powder
- ½ teaspoon baking soda
- ½ tablespoon Celtic sea salt
- 12 tablespoons (1½ sticks) organic butter, cold
- ½ cup chopped roasted macadamia nuts
- ¾ cup organic milk
- 1 tablespoon apple cider vinegar
- Melted dark chocolate (for drizzling)

DIRECTIONS:

1. Preheat oven to 375°F. Line a baking sheet with parchment paper.
2. In a food processor, combine flour, sugar, baking powder, baking soda, and salt. Pulse to blend.
3. Add cold butter and pulse until crumbly.
4. Add chopped macadamia nuts and pulse briefly.
5. In a small bowl, mix milk with apple cider vinegar. Let sit for at least 5 minutes.
6. Add milk mixture to food processor and pulse until dough forms.
7. Turn dough onto a floured sheet of parchment paper.
8. Gently shape into a 10–12 inch circle. Cut into 8 triangles.
9. Bake for 17 minutes, or until lightly golden.
10. Drizzle cooled scones with melted dark chocolate. Cool.

REAL LIFE TIP:

Flash freeze to solidify chocolate before storing in individual serving plastic bags. Put scones in freezer. Ready to eat wholesome pastries.

CHICKEN BONE BROTH

Real food. Deep minerals. Long-term strength.

This is the recipe I use in a 30-quart stock pot. It makes a mineral-rich, collagen-packed broth that we freeze in 16-ounce containers and use year-round as a base for soups, stews, or just as a warm daily tonic.

INGREDIENTS:
- 14 pounds chicken parts (necks, feet, wings—high-collagen cuts)
- 5–6 carrots, chopped
- 4–5 celery stalks, chopped
- 1 bunch fresh parsley
- 1 tablespoon Celtic sea salt
- 1 tablespoon whole black peppercorns
- ½ cup raw
- 6 gallons filtered water

DIRECTIONS:
1. Add all ingredients to a 30-quart stock pot.
2. Bring to a gentle simmer over medium heat.
3. Reduce heat and cook covered for 12 to 24 hours.
4. Once cooled, strain the broth through a fine mesh strainer.
5. Pour into 16-ounce plastic containers, leaving room at the top for expansion.
6. Label and freeze.

REAL LIFE TIP:
The longer it simmers, the richer and more gelatinous it becomes. Your body will feel the difference.

SHORTBREAD WITH PRESERVES

Simple. Real. Unapologetically delicious.

This recipe delivers the kind of sweetness you can stand behind—no fillers, no shortcuts. Just real butter, clean ingredients, and a classic finish.

INGREDIENTS:
- ▸ 2 sticks organic butter, room temperature
- ▸ 2 cups organic flour
- ▸ ½ cup organic sugar
- ▸ ¼ teaspoon Celtic sea salt
- ▸ 12 oz jar of preserves (any flavor or combination)

DIRECTIONS:
1. Preheat oven to 375°F.
2. Line a 9x13-inch baking dish with parchment paper. I use clips on the sides to keep it in place.
3. In a large bowl, mix flour, sugar, and salt.
4. Add butter and work it in with your fingers until the dough resembles coarse crumbs.
5. Press the mixture firmly into the prepared dish to form an even crust.
6. Bake for 15 minutes.
7. Remove from oven and let cool for 2 minutes.
8. Spread the preserves evenly over the crust.
9. Return to oven and bake for an additional 20 minutes.
10. Cool on a rack. Once fully cooled, slice into 12 to 24 pieces, depending on how generous you feel.

REAL LIFE TIP:
Cut into individual servings and freeze in plastic sandwich bags. Great for quick, homemade treats without the mess or the wait.

LEMON TART PIE CRUST

A flaky, real-ingredient crust that holds up beautifully for lemon tarts or any clean dessert.

INGREDIENTS:
- 1 cup all-purpose flour
- 1 stick (½ cup) butter, cold
- 1 egg
- 1 tablespoon heavy cream
- 1 tablespoon apple cider vinegar
- 1 tablespoon organic sugar
- ¼ teaspoon salt

DIRECTIONS:
1. In a mixing bowl, cut cold butter into flour using a fork or pastry cutter until crumbly.
2. Add egg, heavy cream, vinegar, sugar, and salt. Mix gently by hand until dough forms.
3. Roll out on a lightly floured surface and place into a pie tin.
4. Poke the bottom with a fork to prevent bubbling.
5. Bake at 350°F for 23 minutes until lightly golden.
6. Best used the same day for optimal texture.

REAL LIFE TIP:
This crust has structure and flavor—no fillers, no shortcuts. Perfect for lemon tarts, fruit pies, or clean custards.

Real citrus. Real tart. Real good.

LEMON PIE TART

Bright, buttery, and freezer-friendly. This one always disappears fast.

INGREDIENTS:
- ½ cup lemon juice, freshly squeezed
- Zest of 1 lemon
- 4 organic eggs
- ⅔ cup organic sugar
- ¼ teaspoon Celtic sea salt
- 6 tablespoons organic butter
- 1 pre-baked homemade 9-inch crust

DIRECTIONS:
1. In a small saucepan, heat the lemon juice and zest over medium heat until just simmering. Remove from heat.
2. In a separate bowl, whisk the eggs, sugar, and salt until well combined.
3. Slowly pour the egg mixture into the lemon juice, stirring constantly to avoid curdling.
4. Return the pan to medium-low heat. Stir non-stop with a rubber spatula for about 8 minutes, or until the mixture thickens into a smooth custard.
5. Add the butter and stir until completely melted and incorporated.
6. Pour the lemon filling into the pre-baked crust and smooth the top.
7. Chill in the fridge for 2–3 hours, or place in the freezer to set more quickly.
8. Slice and enjoy.

REAL LIFE TIP:
This tart freezes beautifully. Cut into individual servings and store in plastic sandwich bags. Defrost the morning of—no one will know it wasn't freshly made.

PECAN PIE CRUST

Rich, flaky, and built for clean indulgence.

INGREDIENTS:
- 1 cup all-purpose flour
- 1 stick (½ cup) cold butter
- 1 egg
- 1 tablespoon heavy cream
- ¼ teaspoon salt
- 1 teaspoon cold water (only if needed)

DIRECTIONS:
1. In a mixing bowl, cut the cold butter into the flour using a fork or pastry cutter until the mixture is crumbly.
2. Add the egg, heavy cream, and salt. Mix gently by hand until the dough comes together.
3. If it feels too dry, add a teaspoon of cold water.
4. Roll out on a lightly floured surface and press into a 9-inch pie tin.
5. Poke the bottom with a fork to prevent bubbling during baking.
6. Ready to be filled with your pecan pie mixture.

REAL LIFE TIP:
This crust is rich, buttery, and forgiving—perfect for pies that deserve a golden, flaky finish without added fillers or fuss.

Real crust. Real comfort. Real pie.

PECAN PIE

Classic comfort - with a golden top and a scoop of vanilla on the side.

INGREDIENTS:
- 1 cup organic light brown sugar
- ½ cup organic granulated sugar
- 3 large eggs
- 1 cup chopped pecans
- 1 stick butter, melted
- 2 tablespoons organic milk
- 1 tablespoon organic flour
- 1 teaspoon vanilla extract
- 1 unbaked 9-inch homemade pie crust
- 1 cup pecan halves (for topping)
- Vanilla ice cream (for serving)

DIRECTIONS:
1. Preheat oven to 325°F.
2. In a large bowl, mix brown sugar, granulated sugar, and eggs by hand until smooth and creamy.
3. Add chopped pecans, melted butter, milk, flour, and vanilla. Stir to combine.
4. Pour filling into the unbaked pie crust.
5. Arrange pecan halves in a single layer across the top.
6. Bake for 55 minutes, or until the pie is set with a slight jiggle in the center.
7. Let cool before slicing. Serve warm with a scoop of vanilla ice cream.

REAL LIFE TIP:
This pie is rich, buttery, and deeply satisfying—everything a real dessert should be. Keep it classic or freeze slices individually for a no-effort future treat.

TORTILLAS

Soft, foldable, and made from real ingredients—these never last long at our table.

INGREDIENTS:
- 3 cups organic unbleached all-purpose flour
- 1½ teaspoons baking powder
- 1½ teaspoons Celtic sea salt
- ¼ cup olive oil
- 1 cup warm to hot water

DIRECTIONS:
1. In a large bowl, whisk together the flour, baking powder, and salt.
2. Add the olive oil and mix with your fingers until crumbly.
3. Slowly add most of the warm water, mixing by hand to form a dough. Add more water as needed to bring the dough together.
4. Knead for a few minutes until smooth. Shape into a ball.
5. Divide into 12 golf ball–sized portions and cover with plastic wrap until ready to use.
6. Preheat an ungreased cast iron griddle over medium heat.
7. Roll out each ball on a lightly floured surface into a thin round.
8. Place on the hot griddle and cook for 30 seconds per side, flipping with a plastic spatula.
9. Tap with spatula to encourage air bubbles. Remove once lightly golden.

REAL LIFE TIP:
These store well in the fridge or freezer—just warm them in the oven to bring them back to life. Once you've had homemade tortillas, there's no going back.

BUTTER CAKE

Rich, golden, and made with real butter—this one always disappears fast.

INGREDIENTS:
- 3 sticks organic butter (room temperature)
- 1 cup organic granulated sugar
- 6 large organic eggs (room temperature)
- 2½ teaspoons baking powder
- 1½ teaspoons Celtic sea salt
- 3 cups organic all-purpose flour
- 1½ teaspoons vanilla extract
- ¾ cup organic milk mixed with 1 tablespoon apple cider vinegar (let sit 5 minutes to curdle)

DIRECTIONS:
1. Preheat oven to 350°F.
2. In a mixing bowl, beat the butter and sugar together until light and creamy.
3. In a separate bowl, whisk together the flour, baking powder, and salt.
4. Add the first 3 eggs one at a time, mixing after each addition.
5. Add the next 3 eggs, alternating with 2 tablespoons of flour between each one.
6. Stir in the vanilla.
7. Add the remaining flour and milk, alternating between the two until fully incorporated.
8. Pour the batter into a butter-greased Bundt pan.
9. Bake for 45–60 minutes, until golden and a toothpick comes out clean.
10. Cool slightly, then dust with powdered sugar before serving.

REAL LIFE TIP

This cake is even better the next day. Slice and freeze individual servings for a homemade treat any time. Dust with powdered sugar.

PANCAKES

Plump, golden, and made from real ingredients—this is the only pancake recipe I use.

INGREDIENTS:
- ¾ cup organic flour
- ¾ cup organic cake flour
- 1 tablespoon organic sugar
- 1 tablespoon baking powder
- ¼ teaspoon Celtic sea salt
- 1 organic egg
- ¾ cup organic milk mixed with 1 tablespoon apple cider vinegar (let sit 5 minutes to curdle)
- Dash of vanilla extract
- 1 tablespoon organic butter, melted

DIRECTIONS:
1. In a small bowl, combine the milk and apple cider vinegar to make a quick homemade buttermilk. Let it sit for 5 minutes.
2. Melt the butter and set aside.
3. In a large bowl, mix all dry ingredients: flours, sugar, baking powder, and salt.
4. Add the vanilla to the buttermilk mixture.
5. Combine wet and dry ingredients. Add in the egg and melted butter. Mix gently—don't overmix.
6. Set a timer for 5 minutes to let the batter rest while you pre-heat a dry pan over medium heat.
7. Pour batter into the pan to form 4–5 inch pancakes.
8. Flip after 2–3 minutes, cook the other side 2 minutes more, until golden and cooked through.
9. Should yield about 8 plump pancakes.

REAL LIFE TIP:
These freeze beautifully. Store individual pancakes in sandwich bags for quick breakfasts that feel like a treat.

RESOURCES & REFERENCES

T his book is built on lived experience—what I've personally tried, tested, and trusted. While many of the strategies I share are rooted in common sense and ancestral wisdom, I've also pulled inspiration, information, and support from the following books, websites, and products over the years. These resources aren't just citations—they're part of the foundation that helped shape the lifestyle I live and share in these pages.

BOOKS & AUTHORS

These books helped shape my understanding of food, detox, natural healing, and the body's potential to thrive. Each one played a meaningful role in my wellness journey.

- Back to Eden by Jethro Kloss
  A timeless guide to herbs, healing foods, and nature-based remedies.
- Nourishing Traditions by Sally Fallon
  A deep dive into traditional diets, saturated fats, fermentation, and nutrient-dense eating.

- The Fat Flush Plan by Ann Louise Gittleman
  Focused on detox, lymph flow, and supporting the body's fat-burning and cleansing pathways.
- Super Gut by Dr. William Davis
  Explores the powerful connection between gut health, brain clarity, and immune function.
- Iodine: Why You Need It and Can't Live Without It by Dr. David Brownstein
  An essential resource for understanding iodine's role in thyroid health, detoxification, and hormone balance.
- Toxic Superfoods by Sally K. Norton
  A groundbreaking look at dietary oxalates—what they are, how they cause damage, and how removing them can restore energy and reduce inflammation.
- Good Fats Are Good for Women: Menopause by Dr. Elizabeth Bright
  A powerful case for embracing healthy fats during midlife, challenging outdated fat-phobia and restoring hormone balance through ancestral eating.

WEB-BASED RESOURCES

While I prioritize real-world experience over theory, these websites offered helpful context, nutritional insights, and ingredient research throughout my health journey.
- Dr. Berg – drberg.com
  Clear, concise videos on fasting, insulin, liver health, and nutrient timing.
- Organic Facts – organicfacts.net
  Breakdowns of natural remedies, plant benefits, and everyday wellness tips.

- OurHealth – ourhealth.medal.org
  A resource for exploring both mental and physical well-being.
- Cleveland Clinic – my.clevelandclinic.org
  Conventional insights on vitamins, supplements, and body systems.
- Sally K. Norton – sallyknorton.com
  Focused on the effects of dietary oxalates and how they can impact chronic fatigue and inflammation.
- Healthline – healthline.com
  Mainstream explanations of supplements, diets, and wellness strategies.
- WebMD – webmd.com
  Useful for researching symptoms, side effects, and nutrient basics.
- Weston A. Price Foundation – westonaprice.org
  Ancestral food wisdom, fermented traditions, and natural nourishment principles.
- Dr. Clark – drclark.net
  Dr. Hulda Clark's parasite cleanse protocols and detox tools.
- MyBioHack – mybiohack.com
  Insights on brain health, longevity, and simple biohacks for better daily function.
- Dr. David Brownstein – drbrownstein.com
  Supplement insights, thyroid care, and iodine protocols from a holistic MD.
- Eliz Bright, D.C. – elizbright.com
  Carnivore-friendly chiropractic and nutrition support from a wellness-based perspective.
- Happy Mammoth – happymammoth.com
  Supplements designed to support hormones, digestion, and women's health.

BRANDS & PRODUCT SOURCES

These are products and companies I've personally used and continue to trust. They align with my standards for purity, simplicity, and ingredient transparency. I'm not affiliated with these brands—I'm simply sharing what's worked for me.

- Celtic Sea Salt – celticseasalt.com
  Unrefined, mineral-rich salt I use for seasoning, hydration, and detox soaks.
- Dr. Dave's Primal Essence – ddprimalessence.com
  Clean, handcrafted castor oil and tallow-based skincare products.
- California Olive Ranch – californiaoliveranch.com
  Cold-pressed olive oil from California, great for both cooking and finishing.
- Eclectic Herb – eclecticherb.com
  Clean tinctures and herbal support products made with traditional wisdom.
- Earthing – earthing.com
  Grounding mats, bands, and products that reconnect the body to the earth's energy.
- Emerald Labs – emeraldlabs.com
  Additive-free supplements without magnesium stearate or fillers.
- Fatworks – fatworks.com
  Rendered animal fats like tallow, duck fat, and lard—great for cooking and skin.
- General's Hot Sauce – generalshotsauce.com
  Small-batch, American-grown hot sauces with no additives or preservatives.
- NOW Foods – nowfoods.com
  Budget-friendly oils and supplements, great for beginners seeking transparency.

- Oregon's Wild Harvest – oregonswildharvest.com
  Organic herbal formulas and capsules with integrity and care.
- Organic Valley – organicvalley.coop
  Pasture-raised, organic dairy products from a long-trusted cooperative.
- SafeSleeve – safesleevecases.com
  EMF-reducing phone and tablet cases for added tech protection.
- Spices Inc. – spicesinc.com
  A go-to for clean, high-quality spices and blends without hidden additives.
- Straus Family Creamery – strausfamilycreamery.com
  Clean, organic milk, butter, and cream from a regenerative family farm.
- Thorne – thorne.com
  High-purity supplements, used selectively for targeted support.
- Vital Farms – vitalfarms.com
  Ethical, pasture-raised eggs and butter widely available in stores.

FINAL THOUGHTS

Everything in this book comes from real-life use—not theory or trend. These resources supported my own path, and I hope they empower you to ask better questions, seek cleaner options, and find what truly works for your body. Let this list be a launchpad for your own discovery, not a rulebook.

ABOUT THE AUTHOR

Curious by nature, Jackleine Spring explores the deeper side of daily life — where sensation, reflection, and real-world truth intersect.

Jackleine Spring is a natural health enthusiast and wellness strategist who shares first-hand, time-tested approaches for aging well and living with vitality. Her health journey has been shaped by decades of experimentation, real results, and a deep commitment to natural living.

Healthy is beautiful. Aging well is the goal. This book reflects the practical tools and lifestyle shifts that have worked for her—and a few that haven't. From food and supplements to skincare, detox, and mental clarity, every strategy comes from personal experience.

Jackleine lives with her husband and two vibrant 16-year-old dogs—who also benefit from a real food, non-processed lifestyle. Their shared routines, meals, and wellness practices are a testament to how clean living can support longevity across the board.

It's anecdotal. It's honest. And it's all real.

solidgroundhousepublishing.com

Books@solidgroundhousepublishing.com

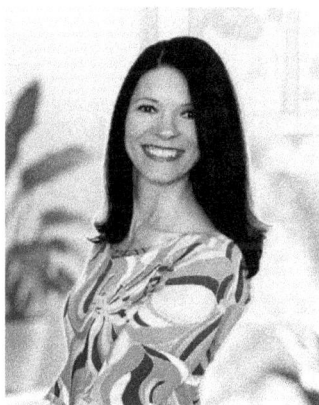

STAY CONNECTED

I f you've enjoyed the strategies in this book and want to keep learning more, you can sign up for occasional health updates, future book announcements, and bonus tips straight from my kitchen.

JOIN THE EMAIL

JOIN.SOLIDGROUNDHOUSEPUBLISHING.COM
Stay in the loop for exclusive updates and tools for living vibrantly and aging gracefully—real strategies, just like the ones you've read in this book.

WANT TO SEE SOME OF THESE RECIPES IN ACTION?
You can check out my YouTube channel, where I quietly demonstrate a few of my real-life power drinks, detox blends, and recipe routines.

Jackleine Spring
https://youtube.com/@spicerack1180

No voiceovers. No fluff. Just a real look at how I prep these strategies in everyday life.

www.ingramcontent.com/pod-product-compliance
Lightning Source LLC
Chambersburg PA
CBHW040830300326

41914CB00084B/2067/J